Best Way To Lose Weight

Your Step-By-Step Guide To Lose Weight In a Month: The Guerrilla Diet Way

By Galit Goldfarb

Table of Contents

Table of Contents 3

Section 1 Dietary Guidelines 9

Introduction 11
Before We Begin 13
The Visualization Technique 15
About the program: 19
Let's Begin: 29
Shopping List 31
Day 1 37
Day 2 39
Day 3 41
Day 4 43
Day 5 45
Day 6 47
Day 7 49
Day 8 51
Day 9 53
Day 10 55
Day 11 57
Day 12 61

Day 13 63
Day 14 65
Day 15 67
Day 16 69
Day 17 73
Day 18 75
Day 19 77
Day 20 79
Day 21 81
Day 22 87
Day 23 89
Day 24 91
Day 25 93
Day 26 99
Day 27 101
Day 28 103
Day 29 105
Day 30 107
To Sum Up: 109

Section 2 Recipes 111
BEST RECIPES FOR HEALTH AND WEIGHT LOSS 113

Lunch & Dinner 115

1. Lentil Soup 117
2. Carrot and Celery Soup.. 119
3. Stir Fry Tofu, Mushroom Combination and Vegetables.. 121
4. Brown Rice and Lentil Stuffed Tomato Cups............ 125
5. Couscous With Chick Pea and Vegetable Soup 129
6. Vegan Soup Stock.. 133
7. Vegan Bean Soup 135
8. Brown Lentil Stew 137
9. Special Green Lentils with Chard or Bok Choy 139
10. Mediterranean Fava Bean Dish 141
11. Home-made Hummus 143
12. Red Lentil Soup.. 145
13. Luscious Tomato Sauce with Peas and Spinach ... 147
14. Sprouted Black Lentil Soup.................................... 151
15. Mediterranean Salad 153
16. Tahini Spread 155
17. Mung Beans and Spinach Stew 157
18. Brown Rice Risotto With Asparagus 159
19. Whole Wheat Pasta with Cauliflower and Nut Sauce .. 161
20. Quinoa, Red Lentil and Wheat Groat Mix 165

21. Buckwheat Noodles with Snow Peas and Asparagus.. 167

22. Whole wheat Rice Noodles with Bean Sprouts and Shelled Edamame 169

23. Tofu and Vegetable Bake 171

24. Cannellini Beans With Olives................................173

25. Vegan Sushi With Whole Grain Rice......................175

26. Aubergine Salad 177

27. Broad Beans with Artichokes 179

28. White Beans with Zucchini....................................183

29. Green Beans and New Potatoes...........................185

30. Black Beans and Pasta...187

31. Cannellini, Aubergine and Sweet Potato Ragout...189

32. White Wine Roasted Potatoes, Peas and Kale......191

33. Potatoes with Asparagus Au Gratin.......................193

34. Mashed Potatoes with Spinach Served with Corn on the Cob...195

35. Red Bean Jambalaya..197

36. Tri Colored Rice Paella 199

37. Quinoa, Mexican Style 201

38. Spaghetti and Tofu Sauce 203

39. Penne with Pine Kernel Cream Sauce...................205

40. Spaghetti and "Meat" Balls....................................207

41. Millet Burger 211
42. Mediterranean Burger 213
43. Lady Fingers and Tofu..215

Breakfast...217

44. Healthy Pancakes 219
45. Tofu Shakshuka..221
46. Porridge...223
47. Oat and Seed Breakfast...225
48. Green Smoothie 227
49. "Milk" Shake 229

Basics..231

50. Brown Rice/Barley..233
51. Brown Rice with Black Lentils 235

Deserts..237

52. Healthy Vegan Winter Carrot Cake........................239

Bread 247

54. Yeast Free Wholemeal Spelt & Walnut Bread........249

Bonus Recipes 253

55. Jerusalem Artichoke...255
56. Miso Soup 257

57. Healthy Vegan Cholent Stew 261
58. Mushrooms Stuffed With Macadamia Creme 265
59. Quinoa Patties..267
60. Vegan Banana Muffins 269
61. Tomato Soup 273
62. Healthy Vegan Birthday Chocolate Cake...............277
63. Healthy Wholegrain Vegan Pizza...........................281
64. Healthy Vegan Apple Crumble 285
65. Healthy Vegan Energy Roll 287
66. Lady Fingers and Chickpea Stew 291
Notes..293
All Books By Galit Goldfarb...303

Section 1

Dietary Guidelines

Introduction

Introducing The Step By Step Guide To Lose Weight In A Month - The Guerrilla Diet & Lifestyle Way: This weight loss program will guide you at the beginning of your weight loss attempt towards creating a healthier life and future for yourself and your family.
By following this program, you will gradually form new lifestyle habits that will stick with you for good. This program is gradual and fulfils your nutritional needs thus it won't overwhelm you or trigger your reptilian brain to fight against your efforts due to your survival instinct coming into play. By following this step-by-step, day-by-day monthly weight loss plan, you will find that, slowly but surely, you will be removing the negative lifestyle habits that perhaps have been giving you short term gratification, but, in the long run, are leading to your self-destruction.
  By following this program, you will be placing your attention on your new lifestyle habits rather than on the results. This will ensure that your new habits will take a

regular place in your life, allowing you to gradually transform negative habits with life-promoting habits instead.

You will also focus on the actions to be taken. Thus, fear from the unknown and fear of not reaching your end result, which is probably way out of your comfort zone, do not come into the equation. Fear is not felt and you feel more in control of your destiny. This program will help you to reach your goals in a more relaxed and controlled way, ensuring lasting effects.

Before We Begin

Before we begin the precise guidelines for losing weight in a month, it is important to understand the basic mindset of losing weight in a month. The mindset of losing weight is success oriented and includes getting into a mode of action. A successful mode of action requires us to create precise goals so that we know exactly where we are going. If you don't know where you are going, you will certainly not reach the destination you desire. This is the reason why goals and plans are so important. This monthly weight loss plan will form your daily goals. However, for you to follow through with your goals you will need to have the groundwork ready. The groundwork which needs to be set BEFORE starting is making sure that you have all of the requirements handy in your kitchen BEFORE you begin with the program. You will need to go shopping and buy all of the required ingredients at your local health food supermarket or farmers market.

I have supplied you with a shopping list that lists everything you will need in order to succeed. (If there are recommended dishes that you know you will not favor and prefer not to have them as part of your diet, just ignore them and choose another dish from another day instead).

Before we begin

In order to succeed you must also have an environment that is supportive for your success, and this means that you should avoid distractions in your near environment that may set you off course. So the next action step to take is to eliminate any distractions you may have in your immediate environment that may keep you from achieving your desire, for example, if your freezer is filled with ice cream and your cupboards are filled with cakes and crips, these will distract you on your path to health and weight loss so it is time to eliminate them before you begin on this program. Remove everything that has no value for where you desire to be in life.

Now that we have dealt with the physical actions to move you closer to your desires, you are now ready to deal with the mental actions for your success.

There is great importance in getting into a success mindset in order for your efforts to fulfill your desire. Therefore, I would like you to begin each day by focusing your attention on your end result. You may do this by following this daily visualization technique:

The Visualization Technique

Reserve a daily time and place where you know that you will not be disturbed for at least five - fifteen minutes. Usually first thing in the morning, and before going off to sleep at night.
Close your eyes.
Take a slow, deep breath in.
Visualize a picture of yourself living with the end result of your desire, be it reaching a very specific desired weight and doing things that you will be doing once this goal is achieved, or just visualize yourself radiating with the health you want to achieve, doing a task you would love to do, or getting into the clothes you would love to see yourself wear. As you visualize this happening, announce repeatedly to your subconscious mind the goal that you are planning to reach.

It is important to understand that avoiding discomfort is the top priority of your reptilian brain. Therefore, your goal must provide you with great pleasure once achieved, and your goal must be attractive enough for you to overwhelm your reptilian brain programming to keep you on the right path towards achieving your goal.

Hold the visualization and the repeated thoughts of your goal for as long as you can until you are either distracted by another competing thought or the picture slowly fades away or changes form. Now do it again.

Do this technique repeatedly, at least once a day, preferably twice, and it will help you make your goal your reality because *focus equals power*.

If you really find it hard to visualize the end result picture in your mind, don't worry. Instead, write down your goal and read it to yourself over and over during the day, every day with passion. Feel as if you have achieved your goals while you are reading them.

I would also suggest reading your daily plan for the following day before going to sleep so that you will be well prepared and ready for the next day. This will not only give you feelings of being in control over your situation, but it will also ensure you have what you need to begin the day. Feelings of control increase self-esteem and give you the energy, courage, and encouragement to go after the fulfillment of your goals with persistence no matter what the current situation seems to be.

Write your goal clearly on a sticky note in several copies and in wording that suggests that you have already achieved the goal. For example: "I weigh 130 pounds or

60 kg.; I am radiating with good health; I look and feel great; I am so happy and grateful" Hang these sticky notes wherever you can see them several times a day, including on your bathroom mirror so you see it first thing in the morning. Include them on the dashboard of your car and on your computer screen.

Focus your mind for a minute or two on the final outcome when you read your goal during the day and flood yourself with feelings that you have already achieved your goals.

Now you have the right mindset to begin. You will undoubtedly reach your goal if you focus your attention on it and on the small daily steps provided in this plan which are needed to get you there.

About the program:

Regarding Your Nutritional and Lifestyle Habits

We will be reducing your empty calorie intake to a minimum to kick start your weight loss. The Guerrilla Diet one month program will guide you using these five simple steps:

(a) You will substitute your processed (white) carbohydrates found in bread/pasta/rice, for whole meal versions. Refined carbohydrates are unnaturally processed foods. They lead to rapid spikes in blood sugar levels which lead to insulin resistance and weight gain. The rapid absorption of glucose after consuming refined carbohydrates induces a sequence of hormonal and metabolic changes that promote excessive food intake. These foods actually increase appetite because the body is hungering for nutrients which it doesn't receive form these processed versions. You will also reduce plain sugar consumption to an absolute minimum. No plain sugar is included in this meal plan.

About the program

You may include chocolate made with a minimum of 85% cocoa, milk free if you have a real urge for chocolate. You may use sugar substitutes including Sweetleaf and Truvia, which come from the stevia plant. These are the best sugar substitutes. Stevia comes from a herb found in Central and South America that is up to 40 times sweeter than sugar but has zero calories and doesn't affect blood sugar levels. Stevia has a bitter aftertaste, but SweetLeaf and Truvia have solved this problem by using the sweetest parts of the stevia plant in their products. By removing sugar from your diet, you will increase your dietary nutrient levels which will help you to avoid food cravings.

(b) You will substitute all dairy products with lentils or beans to reduce saturated fats and the risk for nutrient deficits they lead to in all populations. Lentils are an excellent source of minerals. They are also rich in dietary soluble finer which helps stabilize blood sugar levels, especially important if you suffer from insulin resistance, hypoglycaemia, or diabetes. Lentils are also rich in insoluble fiber which helps balance blood sugar levels by providing a slow and steady energy source. Lentils are also rich in copper, phosphorus, and manganese, and have high levels of iron, protein, vitamin B1, pantothenic acid, zinc, potassium, and vitamin B6. Lentils are rich in complex carbohydrates,

About the program

sodium, fatty acids, and protein, and are therefore a very highly recommended food source. Beans are similar to lentils, but are slightly higher in fiber and slightly lower in minerals yet are also a highly recommended food source. There are so many types of lentils and beans to add variety to your diet and diversity to your nutrient consumption. By consuming lentils and beans, you will no doubt quickly remove any cravings to consume dairy products, help yourself easily and quickly lose weight, and feel good more than you imagine. Sprouting, which increases the availability of minerals, vitamins, and enzymes in the food will also help remove dairy product cravings.

(c) You will substitute half of your meat products with vegetables raw or cooked and non-roasted nuts and seeds (meaning if you currently consume 1000 grams - [35 oz] of meat per week, you will now substitute half of if with more vegetable products and non-roasted nuts and seeds). Animal products switch on genes which increase visceral fat storage (in your belly) which raise the risk for modern Western world chronic diseases and keep you overweight. (Note: Saturated fat also activates genes that increase inflammation while turning off cancer-fighting genes at the same time).

About the program

(d) You will substitute unnatural foods with natural foods. Processed foods with high levels of sugar or fructose, corn syrup, fat, and salt which, when consumed in excess, are seriously harmful to our health. We are evolutionarily inclined to love these foods because their constituents are necessary for survival. These constituents are naturally found in fruits and vegetables. The food industry knows this inclination of ours and spends massive resources on making foods as palatable and as addictive as possible. Therefore, we will need to remove these foods completely from our diet to ensure we regain control of our eating habits. In the beginning, you may feel that foods are too tasteless for you to enjoy because your taste buds have become used to the strong unnatural chemical flavors. To overcome this first period with as little cravings as possible, naturally increase salt rich vegetables to your meals. Salt-rich vegetables include celery, parsley, nori, seaweed, sage, kale, garlic, onion, and other sea vegetables.

(e) You will add walking and exercise blocks into your schedule to increase your metabolism. By increasing physical activity levels, the health risks of obesity and other common modern world diseases are drastically reduced. The importance of physical activity on our health is unwavering. During the recommended thirty-minute exercise blocks, you can do any preferred endurance exercise like walking, biking, or swimming for a minimum of thirty minutes straight. Continuously and uninterruptedly walk around the mall during off-peak hours if unable to walk outside, find a local school track, go to your local park if the weather is fine, or you can choose to ride a bike to work. Any endurance exercise you do continuously for more than thirty minutes once a week is good. Try to fit it within your schedule to make it easier to adopt this practice. If you know that you will not have time to exercise after work, go walking with a coworker at lunch. If a continuous thirty-minute walk seems boring to you, take your smartphone along with you so you can listen to interesting podcasts or music to make this time enjoyable for you. I suggest recording your progress using an activity journal. This will help keep you focused, and also allows you to catch slip-ups in your schedule. I use the "Health" app given for free in every iPhone 5 and subsequent models. This can be one of your most important tools for staying on a healthy path.

Regarding Beverages

You will reduce soft drinks to a minimum or preferably completely remove them from your diet, and focus on only drinking pure water, sparkling (carbonated) water, natural caffeine-free teas or ground coffee this week.
When drinking water, rather than any other beverage, you satisfy your water needs without adding any energy in the form of calories to your diet, and without adding chemicals in the form of artificial sweeteners. Drinking water is also the healthier alternative because it does not change its osmolality and has no glycemic index unlike sugar and artificially sweetened beverages which directly affect blood sugar levels. Drinking water when hungry also makes you feel satiated.

Furthermore, water is a beneficial anti-aging nutrient allowing sufficient hydration which keeps the skin in good health and looking good. Also, any excess water consumed is always safely excreted by the kidneys.

Water removes waste products from our cells and transports important nutrients into them. Water cleanses and rids our body of toxins. It prevents kidney stone formation and constipation and keeps our body functioning at its best.

Regarding Breakfast

First thing in the morning squeeze one whole, (or half), of a lemon into a cup and drink it in one shot. This ritual reduces hunger almost completely and as a bonus will make you completely forget what a sore throat ever felt like.

Following the lemon juice ritual, drink as many glasses of water as you need to feel rehydrated.

Breakfast is a very important meal and through my personal experience and my extensive studies in the field of nutrition, I recommend eating breakfast only when you start to feel hungry in the morning and not earlier. This is why breakfast should be easy and quick to prepare. Once you start feeling hungry, breakfast should be available for you within minutes so that you do not find yourself grabbing an unhealthy alternative just because you are too hungry to wait until something finishes cooking. The moment you start to feel hungry, eat the breakfast that you prepared earlier. The idea is to maintain a healthy blood sugar level without too many spikes, therefore it is important to begin the day with a carbohydrate-rich meal with plenty of fiber.

Regarding Lunch and Dinner

Regarding lunch and dinner, try to add to each meal a side dish of cut vegetables (cucumbers, tomatoes, bell pepper and even onion). Preferably also have some green leafy type of vegetable as well. Having vegetables that are rich in prebiotics to maintain a healthy gut bacteria composition as a side dish accompanying every meal will help your body reduce fat absorption. You may choose to cover the base of your plate with leafy greens to allow them to gain some flavor from your other foods and a dash of any type of onion or garlic as a spice.

Eat the meals when you are hungry, no matter the time of day. If you feel you need to eat your lunch at 11:30 am, then by all means do so. If you are not hungry at 7:00 pm, then wait to eat your dinner until you do feel hungry, but have it prepared and ready to eat so that when feelings of hunger appear you will have something within easy access to feed on.

Snacks should be eaten between meals. However, if you are feeling very hungry, opt to eat the meal itself, even if a little sooner than usual, to avoid consuming too much foods during snack time.

About the program

Regarding Cooking Times

I know how time-consuming cooking can be and therefore if you cannot dedicate time to cooking everyday, I recommend making one day a week preparation day to make all of the foods to be eaten during the course of the week and freeze the main ingredients. Begin your cooking day the night before to allow all legumes to be soaked for a minimum of 12 hours. All meals can then be packaged in separate containers (BPA free) and frozen for the week to come. Choose the most comfortable day for you to do this. This is a very pleasurable day and you will learn to love being creative with the natural ingredients in this diet. Besides, doing the heavy cooking on one day a week, this also keeps the major tidying down to one day a week. If you are fortunate enough to have a private cook, just offer them the recipes and enjoy your healthy meals.

Regarding Your Exercise Program

We will gradually begin an exercise program that will help you burn 500 extra calories. We will do this by adding specific exercise blocks into your schedule. Make sure you perform these exercise blocks on a regular basis. If you find you cannot perform them at the time suggested, do them at the nearest possible time you can.

About the program

Immediately after exercising, try to eat a meal. Remember that ancient humans were physically active before they found a place to stop and forage. This habit helps replenish muscle glycogen stores and heal muscle tissue more quickly.

Regarding The Recipes

Some versions of this book have the recipes form the last part of this book.

In other versions, all of the recipes for this program are found in my book titled:

50 Best Recipes For Health and Weight Loss - The Guerrilla Diet Way. You can receive this book FREE at the following link:

https://goo.gl/2DKpjZ or
https://galitgoldfarb.leadpages.co/free-recipe-book/

It is important that you get your FREE copy of the recipe book before beginning this program.

Let's Begin:

The Step By Step Guide To Lose Weight In A Month - The Guerrilla Diet & Lifestyle Way:

On the next pages, you will find a precise shopping list. Go and purchase some of these new foods and ingredients so that you will not have any excuse to be feeding yourself healthily.

Good Luck! Lets begin!

Shopping List

GENERAL FOODS

Sugar-free apple sauce (free from synthetic sweeteners)
Sugar-free natural jam (free from synthetic sweeteners)
Almond butter spread
Hazelnut butter spread
Natural non-roasted peanut butter
Tomato paste
Sugar-free natural unfrosted Muesli
Almond/Non-GM Soya/Rice/Oat/Coconut Milk (whichever you prefer)
Whole sesame seed spread
Hummus
Premium seaweed sheets for sushi
Natural Mirin
Horseradish paste for sushi
Olives in salt
Non-dairy yogurt
Sugar-free Bran-flakes
Mustard (Heinz)
Soy sauce (low salt)
Coconut oil
Himalayan salt

Rice wine vinegar
Tomato juice
Black pepper
Cayenne pepper
Chilli peppers
Oregano
Turmeric
Cumin

GRAINS

Brown rice crackers
Buckwheat crackers
Corn tortilla
Whole wheat matzo bread
Dr. Kragg crackers
Whole wheat bread
Whole wheat burger bun
Whole wheat spelt bread
Whole wheat pita bread
Whole wheat bagels
Oats
Spelt flour
Organic corn flour
Whole wheat couscous
Tri-colored whole grain rice
Pasta from corn meal

Pasta from whole wheat durum wheat
Buckwheat noodles
Millet
Quinoa
Tri-colored Quinoa
Pearl barley
Wild rice
Basmati brown rice
Long grain brown rice
Red Indian rice
Round (risotto) brown rice

VEGETABLES

Asparagus
Artichoke bottoms
Aubergine
Avocado
Bamia (Lady fingers)
Cauliflower
Celery
Cucumbers
Ginger
Garlic
Leeks
Mushrooms Shiitake
Mushrooms Button

Onions
Red peppers
Parsley and parsley root
Potatoes
Potatoes for preparing baked potatoes
Red beets
Spinach (fresh or frozen)
Sweet potatoes
Tomatoes
Tomatoes - Cherry

FRUIT

When purchasing fruit, buy only fruit that are in season. These are the fruit you will find most in abundance and at a cheaper price. Also try and purchase local food as best as you can.

Apples
Apricots
Banana
Clementines
Dates
Figs
Oranges
Plums
Pears
Pomegranate

peach
Pineapple or dried 9 pineapple slices
Raspberries
Strawberries
Watermelon

LEGUMES

Peas
Chickpeas
Mung beans
White beans
Brown lentils
Red lentils
Corn on the cob
Red beans
Butter beans
Green beans
Yellow beans
Black eyed peas
Snow peas
Bean sprouts
Shelled Edamame

NUTS

Brazil nuts
Almonds

Hazelnuts
Walnuts
Cashew nuts

SEEDS

Flax
Chia
Pumpkin
Sunflower

SUPPLEMENTS

Moringa leaf capsules
Braley grass tablets
Spirulina tablets

Day 1

Upon wakening:
Perform 5-15 minutes focused attention on your goal by performing the visualization exercise of the "Ideal You" found on page 15.

Drink one shot of freshly squeezed lemon juice from 1/2 lemon, followed by enough water to rehydrate yourself after your night's rest.

Supplements:
Today take two tablets of Spirulina to ensure you are receiving all of the nutrients your body needs and to help reduce food cravings.

Breakfast:
1 whole wheat Pita bread with almond butter and sugar-free natural fruit jam to your liking (sugar and additive free of course). I like to taste and variate with different natural jam flavors, this provides variety to the diet. You can also replace almond butter with any other nut butter. You can buy these products at your nearest health food shop or have them delivered directly to your home from

my online shop **HERE**: http://www.guerrillahealthshop.com

Snack:
Summer – 1 apricot, Winter – 1 apple

Lunch:
1-2 cups of brown rice topped with red lentil soup. See recipe # 12

Snack:
5 - 6 Brazil nuts

Dinner:
Pasta from corn or whole durum wheat with tomato pea and spinach sauce. See recipe # 13 *p.147*

Exercise:
Use the stairs at every opportunity you can today instead of using escalators or elevators.

Day 2

Upon wakening:
Perform 5-15 minutes focused attention on your goal by performing the visualization exercise of the "Ideal You" found on page 15.

Drink enough water to rehydrate yourself after your night's rest.

Supplements:
Today take one capsule of Moringa leaves. This helps to reduce appetite and burn more fat.

Breakfast:
2 cups of sugar-free natural Muesli with almond milk. You can buy these products at your nearest health food shop or have them delivered to your home from my online shop **HERE**: http://www.guerrillahealthshop.com

Snack:
Summer – 1 cup of berries, Winter – 1 clementine

Day 2

Lunch:
Wild and brown rice and small sprouted black lentils served with salad See recipes # 50 & # 14

Snack:
2 carrots dipped in sesame spread.

Dinner:
Whole wheat bread with a plate of natural hummus and oil free fried Shiitake mushrooms. See hummus recipe # 11

Exercise:
Today is your first endurance training day. Power walk (faster than your usual walk), run, swim or bike continuously for 30 minutes at a time most suitable for you.

Day 3

Upon wakening:
Perform 5-15 minutes focused attention on your goal by performing the visualization exercise of the "Ideal You" found on page 15.

Drink one shot of freshly squeezed lemon juice from 1/2 lemon, followed by enough water to rehydrate yourself after your night's rest.

Supplements:
Today take one tablet of Barley Grass to ensure you are receiving all the nutrients your body needs. You can buy this product and everything on this menu at your nearest health food shop or have them delivered to your home from my online shop **HERE**: http://www.guerrillahealthshop.com

Breakfast:
Whole wheat bagel with whole sesame seed paste.

Snack:
Summer – 1 plum, Winter – 1 orange

Day 3

Lunch:
Red Indian rice with mung beans and spinach stew. See recipe # 17

Snack:
5 almonds

Dinner:
Vegan sushi. See recipe # 25

Exercise:
Park your car a little further away from your destinations today so you can take a short power walk.

Day 4

Upon wakening:
Perform 5-15 minutes focused attention on your goal by performing the visualization exercise of the "Ideal You" found on page 15.

Drink enough water to rehydrate yourself after your night's rest.

Supplements:
Today take one capsule of Moringa to reduce appetite and burn fat.

Breakfast:
Whole oats with flax, chia, pumpkin and sunflower seeds with oat milk. You can place the oats, sunflower seeds, pumpkin seeds, chia seeds, flax seeds and raisins in a coffee blending machine (extremely cheap to buy at any hardware shop or on my web store) and grind everything together for 2-4 seconds. Then add milk from either soya, rice, almond, coconut or oats and you're ready to eat. You can buy these products at your nearest health food shop or have them delivered to your home from my online shop **HERE**: http://www.guerrillahealthshop.com

Day 4

Snack:
Summer – 1 cup of strawberries, Winter – pear

Lunch:
Brown round rice risotto and asparagus. See recipe # 18

Snack:
5 hazelnuts

Dinner:
Aubergine salad served with whole wheat bread, olives and tahini or sesame paste. See recipes # 16 and # 26

Exercise:
Take a one hour stroll with a friend or stroll continuously in the shopping mall for one hour.

Day 5

Upon wakening:
Perform 5-15 minutes focused attention on your goal by performing the visualization exercise of the "Ideal You" found on page 15.

Drink one shot of freshly squeezed lemon juice from 1/2 lemon, followed by enough water to rehydrate you after your night's rest.

Breakfast:
Whole wheat toast with avocado sprinkled with sunflower seeds.

Snack:
Summer – 2 figs, Winter – 2 dates

Lunch:
Mexican style quinoa. See recipe # 37

Snack:
Half a handful of raw pumpkin seeds

Day 5

Dinner:
Millet burger. See recipe # 41

Exercise:
Today do 20 Abdominal Curls:
Lie down with your knees bent and your feet placed flat on the ground.
1. Place your hands either behind your head or on opposing shoulders by crossing your hands over your chest.
2. Tighten your abdominal muscles and then slowly lift your head and then your shoulder blades off the floor until you reach a 90-degree angle.
3. Slowly bring your back to the floor in a slightly arched fashion.
4. Repeat.

Day 6

Upon wakening:
Perform 5-15 minutes focused attention on your goal by performing the visualization exercise of the "Ideal You" found on page 15.

Drink enough water to rehydrate you after your night's rest.

Supplements:
Today take one tablet of Spirulina to ensure you are receiving all the nutrients your body needs and to help reduce food cravings.

Breakfast:
Healthy pancakes. See recipe # 39

Snack:
Summer – 1 grapefruit, Winter – 1 nectarine

Lunch:
Megadra served with tahini salad. See recipes # 51 & # 16

Day 6

Snack:
Half a handful of sunflower seeds

Dinner:
Lady fingers and tofu served with whole grain rice. See recipe # 43

Exercise:
Today watch an exercise video and do the exercises in your house along with the video. Here is one I recommend:
https://www.youtube.com/watch?v=FTT4W8ygJ7w

Day 7

Upon wakening:
Perform 5-15 minutes focused attention on your goal by performing the visualization exercise of the "Ideal You" found on page 15.

Drink one shot of freshly squeezed lemon juice from 1/2 lemon, followed by enough water to rehydrate you after your night's rest.

Supplements:
Today take two tablets of Barley Grass to ensure you are receiving all the nutrients your body needs.

Breakfast:
Fruit salad sprinkled with chia and flax seeds.

Snack:
1 Banana

Lunch:
1 Large baked Potato topped with corn served with salad.

Day 7

Snack:
2 dates served with a non-dairy yogurt

Dinner:
Bean soup. See recipe # 7

Exercise:
Take a one-hour evening stroll in the fresh air with a friend if weather permits or inside a shopping mall.

Day 8

Upon wakening:
Perform 5-15 minutes focused attention on your goal by performing the visualization exercise of the "Ideal You" found on page 15.

Drink enough water to rehydrate you after your night's rest.

Breakfast:
Oat and seed breakfast. See recipe # 47. You can buy these products at your nearest health food shop or have them delivered to your home from my online shop **HERE**: http://www.guerrillahealthshop.com

Snack:
Summer – peach, Winter – apple

Lunch:
Red bean jambalaya. See recipe # 36

Snack:
Half a handful of walnuts

Day 8

Dinner:
Potatoes with asparagus au gratin: See recipe # 33

Exercise:
Endurance training day. Power walk (faster than your usual walk), run, swim or bike continuously for 30 minutes.

Day 9

Upon wakening:
Perform 5-15 minutes focused attention on your goal by performing the visualization exercise of the "Ideal You" found on page 15.

Drink one shot of freshly squeezed lemon juice from 1/2 lemon, followed by enough water to rehydrate you after your night's rest.

Supplements:
Today take one capsule of Moringa to reduce appetite and burn fat.

Breakfast:
Milkshake. See recipe # 49

Snack:
Summer – 1 cup of watermelon cubes, Winter – clementine

Lunch:
Black beans and pasta. See recipe # 30

Snack:
1 cup pineapple cubes in season or 3 slices of dried pineapple

Dinner:
Mashed potatoes with artichoke bottoms and broad beans. See recipe # 28

Exercise:
Today, park your car a little further away from your destinations so you can take short power walks throughout the day.

Day 10

Upon wakening:
Perform 5-15 minutes focused attention on your goal by performing the visualization exercise of the "Ideal You" found on page 15.

Drink enough water to rehydrate you after your night's rest.

Supplements:
Today take two tablets of Barley Grass to ensure you are receiving all the nutrients your body needs.

Breakfast:
2 Dr. Kraggs crackers or 1 Whole-wheat matzo with natural peanut butter and sugar-free natural fruit jam. You can buy these products at your nearest health food shop or have them delivered to your home from my online shop **HERE**: http://www.guerrillahealthshop.com

Snack:
1 cup of pomegranate seeds

Day 10

Lunch:
Stuffed tomato cups. See recipe # 4
Snack:
5 cherry tomatoes dipped in sesame spread

Dinner:
Cannellini, aubergine and sweet potato ragout. See recipe # 31

Exercise:
Use the stairs at every opportunity you can today instead of using escalators or elevators.

Day 11

Upon wakening:
Perform 5-15 minutes focused attention on your goal by performing the visualization exercise of the "Ideal You" found on page 15.

Drink one shot of freshly squeezed lemon juice from 1/2 lemon, followed by enough water to rehydrate you after your night's rest.

Supplements:
Today take one tablet of Spirulina to ensure you are receiving all the nutrients your body needs and to help reduce food cravings.

Breakfast:
4 Rice crackers and avocado with sesame paste.

Snack:
Summer –1/2 cup cherries, Winter – pear

Lunch:
Tri-colored rice Paella. See recipe # 36

Day 11

Snack:
5 Almonds

Dinner:
Whole-wheat couscous with chickpea and vegetable soup. See recipe # 5

Exercise:
Today Perform the following three simple strength exercises either in a gym or at home using home barbells or anything that can easily be grasped that weigh 1–6 kg (2–13 pounds) according to your current physical ability. These are whole body workouts working on all major muscle groups.

Perform three sets of ten repetitions each for each of the following three strength exercises. In the first exercise, focus on raising and lowering your weights and holding your body in a controlled manner.

Triceps Press. This exercise works on all three of the triceps muscles, shoulder, abdomen and back stabilizing muscles.
> 1. Get into a plank position with your toes resting on a stair, table, or ball. Place your hands a little closer than shoulder-width apart.

Day 11

2. Bend your arms slowly until your elbows reach a 90-degree angle.
3. Press back up to straighten.
4. Return to starting position and repeat.

Superman. This exercise works the back and bottom gluteus maximus muscles.
1. Lie face down with arms and legs extended, toes pointed, palms down.
2. Inhale while raising arms and legs as high as you can; pause.
3. Exhale while slowly returning to starting position.

Abdominal Curls. This exercise works on your abdominal muscles.
1. Lie down with your knees bent and your feet placed flat on the ground.
2. Place your hands either behind your head or on opposing shoulders by crossing your hands over your chest.
3. Tighten your abdominal muscles and then slowly lift your head and then your shoulder blades off the floor until you reach a 90-degree angle.
4. Slowly bring your back to the floor in a slightly arched fashion.
5. Repeat.

Day 12

Upon wakening:
Perform 5-15 minutes focused attention on your goal by performing the visualization exercise of the "Ideal You" found on page 15.

Drink enough water to rehydrate you after your night's rest.

Breakfast:
Tofu shakshuka. See recipe # 45

Snack:
Summer – 1 apricot, Winter – 1 apple

Lunch:
Mediterranean burger – See recipe served with chopped vegetable salad. See recipe # 42

Snack:
5 hazelnuts

Dinner:
Rice noodles with bean sprouts. See recipe # 22

Day 12

Exercise:
Today watch an exercise video and do the exercises in your house along with the video. Here is a dance workout. https://www.youtube.com/watch?v=ZsVp7wRWG7I

Day 13

Upon wakening:
Perform 5-15 minutes focused attention on your goal by performing the visualization exercise of the "Ideal You" found on page 15.

Drink one shot of freshly squeezed lemon juice from 1/2 lemon, followed by enough water to rehydrate you after your night's rest.

Supplements:
Today take one capsule of Moringa to reduce appetite and burn fat.

Breakfast:
Whole spelt bread with hazelnut butter and apple sauce. You can buy these products at your nearest health food shop or have them delivered to your home from my online shop **HERE**: http://www.guerrillahealthshop.com

Snack:
Summer – 1 cup of berries, Winter – pear

Day 13

Lunch:
Brown lentils with Swiss chard or Bok choy served on Brown basmati rice. See recipe # 9

Snack:
Half a handful of raw pumpkin seeds

Dinner:
Green beans and new potatoes. See recipe # 29

Exercise:
Endurance training day. Power walk (faster than your usual walk), run, swim or bike continuously for 30 minutes.

Day 14

Upon wakening:
Perform 5-15 minutes focused attention on your goal by performing the visualization exercise of the "Ideal You" found on page 15.

Drink enough water to rehydrate you after your night's rest.

Supplements:
Today take two tablets of Barley Grass to ensure you are receiving all the nutrients your body needs.

Breakfast:
2 cups of sugar-free natural Muesli with almond milk.

Snack:
1 cup of pomegranate seeds

Lunch:
Tofu and vegetable bake – See recipe # 23, served on red Indian rice.

Day 14

Snack:
Half a handful of sunflower seeds

Dinner:
Aubergine salad, and whole wheat bread. See recipe # 26

Exercise:
Use the stairs at every opportunity you can today instead of using escalators or elevators.

Day 15

Upon wakening:
Perform 5-15 minutes focused attention on your goal by performing the visualization exercise of the "Ideal You" found on page 15.

Drink one shot of freshly squeezed lemon juice from 1/2 lemon, followed by enough water to rehydrate you after your night's rest.

Supplements:
Today take one tablet of Spirulina to ensure you are receiving all the nutrients your body needs and to help reduce food cravings.

Breakfast:
Wholewheat bagel with sesame paste and sugar-free natural fruit jam.

Snack:
Summer – 1 cup of raspberries, Winter – 1 clementine

Day 15

Lunch:
Quinoa, red lentil and wheat groat tabouli. See recipe # 20

Snack:
2 dates served with a non-dairy yogurt

Dinner:
Buckwheat noodles with stir fried vegetables. See recipe # 21

Exercise:
Take a one-hour evening stroll in the fresh air with a friend if weather permits or inside a shopping mall.

Day 16

Upon wakening:
Perform 5-15 minutes focused attention on your goal by performing the visualization exercise of the "Ideal You" found on page 15.

Drink enough water to rehydrate you after your night's rest.

Breakfast:
Fruit salad sprinkled with chia and flax seeds.

Snack:
Summer – 1 plum, Winter – 1 orange

Lunch:
Fava beans with whole wheat pita bread. See recipe # 10

Snack:
A handful of walnuts

Dinner:
Whole wheat bread with a plate of natural hummus and oil free fried Shiitake mushrooms. See recipe # 11

Day 16

Exercise:
Today Perform the following three simple strength exercises either in a gym or at home using home barbells or anything that can easily be grasped that weigh 1–6 kg (2–13 pounds) according to your current physical ability.

Perform three sets of ten repetitions each for each of the three strength exercises below. In the first exercise focus on raising and lowering your weights and holding your body in a controlled manner.

Triceps Press. This exercise works on all three of the triceps muscles, shoulder, abdomen and back stabilizing muscles.
1. Get into a plank position with your toes resting on a stair, table, or ball. Place your hands a little closer than shoulder-width apart.
2. Bend your arms slowly until your elbows reach a 90-degree angle.
3. Press back up to straighten.
4. Return to starting position and repeat.

Superman. This exercise works the back and bottom gluteus maximus muscles.
1. Lie face down with arms and legs extended, toes pointed, palms down.
2. Inhale while raising arms and legs as high as you can; pause.

Day 16

3. Exhale while slowly returning to starting position.

Abdominal Curls. This exercise works on your abdominal muscles.

1. Lie down with your knees bent and your feet placed flat on the ground.
2. Place your hands either behind your head or on opposing shoulders by crossing your hands over your chest.
3. Tighten your abdominal muscles and then slowly lift your head and then your shoulder blades off the floor until you reach a 90-degree angle.
4. Slowly bring your back to the floor in a slightly arched fashion.
5. Repeat.

Day 17

Upon wakening:
Perform 5-15 minutes focused attention on your goal by performing the visualization exercise of the "Ideal You" found on page 15.

Drink one shot of freshly squeezed lemon juice from 1/2 lemon, followed by enough water to rehydrate you after your night's rest.

Supplements:
Today take one capsule of Moringa to reduce appetite and burn fat.

Breakfast:
Bran-flakes with non-GM soy milk. You can buy these products at your nearest health food shop or have them delivered to your home from my online shop **HERE**: http://www.guerrillahealthshop.com

Snack:
Summer – 1 peach, Winter – 1 apple

Lunch:
Whole wheat pasta with black-beans. See recipe # 30

Dinner:
Vegan sushi. See recipe # 25

Exercise:
Endurance training day. Power walk (faster than your usual walk), run, swim or bike continuously for 30 minutes.

Day 18

Upon wakening:
Perform 5-15 minutes focused attention on your goal by performing the visualization exercise of the "Ideal You" found on page 15.

Drink enough water to rehydrate you after your night's rest.

Supplements:

Today take one tablet of Barley Grass to ensure you are receiving all the nutrients your body needs.

Breakfast:
Corn tortilla with avocado sprinkled with sunflower seeds.

Snack:
Summer – 1 cup of watermelon cubes, Winter – clementine

Lunch:
Lentil soup. See recipe # 1

Day 18

Snack:
2 sliced red peppers dipped in sesame seed spread.

Dinner:
Pasta with cauliflower and nut sauce. See recipe # 19

Exercise:
Today watch an exercise video and do the exercises in your house along with the video. Here is one I recommend doing today using a resistance band:
https://www.youtube.com/watch?v=wm4-r_ON_3A

if you don't have a resistance band, try this workout instead:
https://www.youtube.com/watch?v=3o4aHHXJDBc

Day 19

Upon wakening:
Perform 5-15 minutes focused attention on your goal by performing the visualization exercise of the "Ideal You" found on page 15.

Drink one shot of freshly squeezed lemon juice from 1/2 lemon, followed by enough water to rehydrate you after your night's rest.

Supplements:
Today take one tablet of Spirulina to ensure you are receiving all the nutrients your body needs and to help reduce food cravings.

Breakfast:
Whole oats with flax, chia, pumpkin and sunflower seeds with rice milk. You can buy these products at your nearest health food shop or have them delivered to your home from my online shop **HERE**: http://www.guerrillahealthshop.com

Snack:
Summer – 1 cup of berries, Winter – 1 pear

Day 19

Lunch:
Red bean Jambalaya. See recipe # 35

Snack:
A handful of Almonds

Dinner:
Stir fry tofu and vegetables served with Brown noodles. See recipe # 3

Exercise:
Endurance training day. Power walk (faster than your usual walk), run, swim or bike continuously for 30 minutes.

Day 20

Upon wakening:
Perform 5-15 minutes focused attention on your goal by performing the visualization exercise of the "Ideal You" found on page 15.

Drink enough water to rehydrate you after your night's rest.

Breakfast:
Whole-wheat bagel with sesame paste.

Snack:
1 banana

Lunch:
Bean soup served on wild rice. See recipe # 7

Snack:
A handful of hazelnuts

Dinner:
Wholewheat penne pasta with tomato and pea sauce. See recipe # 13

Day 20

Exercise:
Today, park your car a little further away from your destinations so you can take short power walks throughout the day.

Day 21

Upon wakening:
Perform 5-15 minutes focused attention on your goal by performing the visualization exercise of the "Ideal You" found on page 15.

Drink one shot of freshly squeezed lemon juice from 1/2 lemon, followed by enough water to rehydrate you after your night's rest.

Supplements:
Today take one capsule of Moringa to reduce appetite and burn fat.

Breakfast:
4 Buckwheat crackers and avocado with sesame paste.

Snack:
Summer – 1 plum, Winter – 1 orange

Lunch:
Cannellini and rice served with salad. See recipe # 24

Day 21

Snack:
A handful of raw pumpkin seeds

Dinner:
Mediterranean burger with whole-wheat bun. See recipe # 42

Exercise:
Today Perform the following five simple strength exercises either in a gym or at home using home barbells or anything that can easily be grasped that weigh 1–6 kg (2–13 pounds) according to your current physical ability. These are whole body workouts working on all major muscle groups.
Perform three sets of ten repetitions each for each of the five strength exercises below. Focus on raising and lowering your weights and holding your body in a controlled manner.

> **Squat to Overhead Press.** This exercise works leg quadriceps and hamstring muscles, bottom gluteus maximus muscles, abdominal muscles, and shoulder muscles.
> 1. Hold a hand weight of 1–6 kg (2–13-pound weight) in each hand held at chest height, palms facing forward.

2. Stand with feet shoulder-width apart with elbows bent.
3. Lower into a squat position, making sure your knees do not bend forward over your toe line. Hold for a moment.
4. Straighten your knees to stand up while raising the weights above your head.
5. Return to starting position and repeat.

Step with Bicep Curl. This exercise works leg quadriceps and hamstring muscles, bottom gluteus maximus muscles, abdominal muscles, and hand biceps muscles.

1. Stand with one foot on a sturdy bench or low step, holding a weight in each hand.
2. Lift yourself up to standing on the step. At the same time, curl weights up toward shoulders.
3. Go back down and raise your other leg on the step.
4. Again, lift yourself up to standing on the step. At the same time, curl weights up toward shoulders.
5. Switch sides and repeat.

Triceps Press. This exercise works on all three of the triceps muscles, shoulder, abdomen and back stabilizing muscles.

1. Get into a plank position with your toes resting on a stair, table, or ball. Place your hands a little closer than shoulder-width apart.
2. Bend your arms slowly until your elbows reach a 90-degree angle.
3. Press back up to straighten.
4. Return to starting position and repeat.

Superman. This exercise works the back and bottom gluteus maximus muscles.
1. Lie face down with arms and legs extended, toes pointed, palms down.
2. Inhale while raising arms and legs as high as you can; pause.
3. Exhale while slowly returning to starting position.

Abdominal Curls. This exercise works on your abdominal muscles.
1. Lie down with your knees bent and your feet placed flat on the ground.
2. Place your hands either behind your head or on opposing shoulders by crossing your hands over your chest.
3. Tighten your abdominal muscles and then slowly lift your head and then your shoulder blades off the floor until you reach a 90-degree angle.

Day 21

4. Slowly bring your back to the floor in a slightly arched fashion.
5. Repeat.

Day 22

Upon wakening:
Perform 5-15 minutes focused attention on your goal by performing the visualization exercise of the "Ideal You" found on page 15.

Drink enough water to rehydrate you after your night's rest.

Supplements:
Today take two tablets of Barley Grass to ensure you are receiving all the nutrients your body needs.

Breakfast:
1 whole wheat Pita with almond butter and sugar-free natural fruit jam.

Snack:
1 cup of pomegranate seeds

Lunch:
Brown lentil stew served with whole grain pearl barley. See recipe # 8

Day 22

Snack:
Half a handful of sunflower seeds

Dinner:
Arabic salad served with whole wheat bread, olives and tahini or sesame paste. See recipes # 15 & 16

Exercise:
Take a one-hour evening stroll in the fresh air with a friend if weather permits or inside a shopping mall.

Day 23

Upon wakening:
Perform 5-15 minutes focused attention on your goal by performing the visualization exercise of the "Ideal You" found on page 15.

Drink one shot of freshly squeezed lemon juice from 1/2 lemon, followed by enough water to rehydrate you after your night's rest.

Supplements:
Today take one tablet of Spirulina to ensure you are receiving all the nutrients your body needs and to help reduce food cravings.

Breakfast:
Healthy pancakes. See recipe # 44

Snack:
Summer – 1 apricot, Winter – 1 apple

Lunch:
Quinoa, Mexican style. See recipe # 37.

Day 23

Snack:
2 dates served with a non-dairy yogurt

Dinner:
Spaghetti and "meat balls". See recipe # 40

Exercise:
Today watch an exercise video and do the exercises in your house along with the video. Here is a kickboxing workout:
https://www.youtube.com/watch?v=Vve4BVTZ0QU

Day 24

Upon wakening:
Perform 5-15 minutes focused attention on your goal by performing the visualization exercise of the "Ideal You" found on page 15.

Drink enough water to rehydrate you after your night's rest.

Breakfast:
3 Dr. Kragg crackers or 2 Whole wheat matzo bread with hazelnut butter and 100% fruit jam.

Snack:
Summer – 1 grapefruit, Winter – 1 nectarine

Lunch:
Penne with pine kernel cream sauce. See recipe # 39

Snack:
A handful of walnuts

Day 24

Dinner:

White wine roasted potatoes, peas and kale. See recipe # 32

Exercise:

Endurance training day. Power walk (faster than your usual walk), run, swim or bike continuously for 30 minutes.

Day 25

Upon wakening:
Perform 5-15 minutes focused attention on your goal by performing the visualization exercise of the "Ideal You" found on page 15.

Drink one shot of freshly squeezed lemon juice from 1/2 lemon, followed by enough water to rehydrate you after your night's rest.

Supplements:
Today take one capsule of Moringa to reduce appetite and burn fat.

Breakfast:
Tofu scramble

Snack:
Summer – 1 cup of strawberries, Winter – 1 pear

Lunch:
Lady fingers and tofu. See recipe # 43

Day 25

Snack:
A small handful of Brazil nuts

Dinner:
Magadra served with salad. See recipe # 51

Exercise:
Today I would like you to perform the following five simple strength exercises either in a gym or at home using home barbells or anything that can easily be grasped that weigh 1–6 kg (2–13 pounds) according to your current physical ability. These are whole body workouts working on all major muscle groups.

Perform three sets of ten repetitions each for each of the five strength exercises below. Focus on raising and lowering your weights and holding your body in a controlled manner.

Squat to Overhead Press. This exercise works leg quadriceps and hamstring muscles, bottom gluteus maximus muscles, abdominal muscles, and shoulder muscles.
1. Hold a hand weight of 1–6 kg (2–13-pound weight) in each hand held at chest height, palms facing forward.

Day 25

2. Stand with feet shoulder-width apart with elbows bent.
3. Lower into a squat position, making sure your knees do not bend forward over your toe line. Hold for a moment.
4. Straighten your knees to stand up while raising the weights above your head.
5. Return to starting position and repeat.

Step with Bicep Curl. This exercise works leg quadriceps and hamstring muscles, bottom gluteus maximus muscles, abdominal muscles, and hand biceps muscles.

1. Stand with one foot on a sturdy bench or low step, holding a weight in each hand.
2. Lift yourself up to standing on the step. At the same time, curl weights up toward shoulders.
3. Go back down and raise your other leg on the step.
4. Again, lift yourself up to standing on the step. At the same time, curl weights up toward shoulders.
5. Switch sides and repeat.

Triceps Press. This exercise works on all three of the triceps muscles, shoulder, abdomen and back stabilizing muscles.

1. Get into a plank position with your toes resting on a stair, table, or ball. Place your hands a little closer than shoulder-width apart.
2. Bend your arms slowly until your elbows reach a 90-degree angle.
3. Press back up to straighten.
4. Return to starting position and repeat.

Superman. This exercise works the back and bottom gluteus maximus muscles.
1. Lie face down with arms and legs extended, toes pointed, palms down.
2. Inhale while raising arms and legs as high as you can; pause.
3. Exhale while slowly returning to starting position.

Abdominal Curls. This exercise works on your abdominal muscles.
1. Lie down with your knees bent and your feet placed flat on the ground.
2. Place your hands either behind your head or on opposing shoulders by crossing your hands over your chest.
3. Tighten your abdominal muscles and then slowly lift your head and then your shoulder blades off the floor until you reach a 90-degree angle.

Day 25

4. Slowly bring your back to the floor in a slightly arched fashion.
5. Repeat.

Day 26

Upon wakening:
Perform 5-15 minutes focused attention on your goal by performing the visualization exercise of the "Ideal You" found on page 15.
Drink enough water to rehydrate you after your night's rest.

Supplements:
Today take one tablet of Barley Grass to ensure you are receiving all the nutrients your body needs.

Breakfast:
1 whole wheat Pita with almond butter and sugar-free natural fruit jam.

Snack:
1 Cup of cubed pineapple if in season. Off season, 3 slices of dried pineapple

Lunch:
Stir fry tofu and vegetables served with Brown round rice. See recipe # 22

Day 26

Snack:
2 carrots dipped in sesame seed spread.

Dinner:
Mashed potatoes with spinach and corn. See recipe # 34

Exercise:
Park your car a little further away from your destination so you can take a short power walk.

Day 27

Upon wakening:
Perform 5-15 minutes focused attention on your goal by performing the visualization exercise of the "Ideal You" found on page 15.

Drink one shot of freshly squeezed lemon juice from 1/2 lemon, followed by enough water to rehydrate you after your night's rest.

Supplements:
Today take one tablet of Spirulina to ensure you are receiving all the nutrients your body needs and to help reduce food cravings.

Breakfast:
4 Rice crackers and avocado with sesame paste.

Snack:
Summer – 2 figs, Winter – 2 dates

Lunch:
Whole tri-color Quinoa Tabouli. See recipe # 20

Day 27

Snack:
5 Almonds

Dinner:
Whole-wheat couscous with chickpea and vegetable soup. See recipe # 5

Exercise:
Take a one-hour evening stroll in the fresh air with a friend if weather permits or inside a shopping mall.

Day 28

Upon wakening:
Perform 5-15 minutes focused attention on your goal by performing the visualization exercise of the "Ideal You" found on page 15.

Drink enough water to rehydrate you after your night's rest.

Breakfast:
Corn tortilla with avocado sprinkled with sunflower seeds.

Snack:
Summer – 1 cup of cherries, Winter – apple

Lunch:
Brown rice risotto with asparagus. See recipe # 18

Snack:
Half a handful of hazelnuts

Day 28

Dinner:

Green beans with spinach and new potatoes. See recipe # 29

Exercise:

Today watch an exercise video and do the exercises in your house along with the video. Here is a dance workout. https://www.youtube.com/watch?v=Vve4BVTZ0QU

Day 29

Upon wakening:
Perform 5-15 minutes focused attention on your goal by performing the visualization exercise of the "Ideal You" found on page 15.

Drink one shot of freshly squeezed lemon juice from 1/2 lemon, followed by enough water to rehydrate you after your night's rest.

Supplements:
Today take one capsule of Moringa to reduce appetite and burn fat.

Breakfast:
Whole oats with flax, chia, hazelnuts and dates served with coconut milk. You can buy these products at your nearest health food shop or have them delivered to your home from my online shop **HERE**: http://www.guerrillahealthshop.com

Snack:
Summer – 1 cup of cubed watermelon, Winter – 1 clementine

Day 29

Lunch:
Broad beans with artichokes. See recipe # 27

Snack:
Half a handful of pumpkin seeds

Dinner:
Millet burger. See recipe # 41

Exercise:
Endurance training day. Power walk (faster than your usual walk), run, swim or bike continuously for 30 minutes.

Day 30

Upon wakening:
Perform 5-15 minutes focused attention on your goal by performing the visualization exercise of the "Ideal You" found on page 15.

Drink enough water to rehydrate you after your night's rest.

Supplements:
Today take two tablets of Barley Grass to ensure you are receiving all the nutrients your body needs.

Breakfast:
1 whole wheat Pita with almond butter and sugar-free natural fruit jam.

Snack:
1 cup of pomegranate seeds

Lunch:
Lentil and rice stuffed tomatoes served with salad. See recipe #4

Day 30

Snack:
Half a handful of sunflower seeds

Dinner:
Pasta with cauliflower and nut sauce. See recipe # 19

Exercise:
Take a one-hour evening stroll in the fresh air with a friend if weather permits or inside a shopping mall.

To Sum Up:

Even if you have not lost all of the weight you desired to lose during this month, you will continue to lose all of the weight you desire if you persist with the recommendations in this guide. I promise you that if you just keep at it you will reach your desired weight in due time.

Wishing you the best of luck in becoming happy and healthy.

If you would like personal counseling with this diet, I recommend you join my online training program.
This program is all you will need to create the health you deserve to have.

With this special one time discount code you will receive the course at a 50% off! Just because you have proven that this subject is important for you.

Insert the code below in the "Redeem Coupon" space.

Coupon code: 50offspecial

To sum up

If you would like more information about this course go to this link HERE:
https://goo.gl/hZWRf7

For those of you who have enjoyed the book but prefer an individual touch with small group mentoring calls to get you quickly into the process of losing weight and achieving the health that you deserve for good with added personal touch, I have a group coached programs with only a few participants designed especially for you. These coached programs are offered a few times a year. Please visit **The Guerrilla/ ~~Gorilla~~ Diet and Lifestyle Program** website (www.TheGuerillaDiet.com) to find out when the next coached online program begins.

For those who prefer one-on-one private coaching sessions, please write this down on the "Contact us" form at our website at www.TheGuerillaDiet.com.

For any questions or support, just mail us at: support@theguerrilladiet.com

Or write to us on Facebook:

The Guerrilla Diet Lifestyle Program

Section 2 Recipes

BEST RECIPES FOR HEALTH AND WEIGHT LOSS

THE GUERRILLA DIET WAY

By Galit Goldfarb

Lunch & Dinner

1. Lentil Soup

Great as a winter appetiser that will keep you feeling full and satisfied for hours

Serves: 4
Preparation time: 15 minutes
Cooking time: 1 hour 40 minutes

Ingredients

2 cups brown lentils
1 cup cut carrots
1/2 cup cut potatoes
12 cups water
1/2 tsp himalayan salt
1/2 tsp ground cumin
1/4 tsp all spice
1 medium onion, finely chopped
1 tsp coconut oil
1/4 cup finely chopped fresh parsley

Instructions:

1. Wash lentils, peel and cut potatoes and carrots.
2. Place in a pot with water. Bring to boil. Cover and gently simmer for about 1.5 hours
3. If you wish: transfer soup to a food processor or blender while adding 1 cup of water. Blend well. Put mixture back in pot
4. Simmer over a low heat while adding all spice, cumin and salt.
5. Fry chopped onion till soft or use raw onion.
6. Add onion to lentil mixture. Bring to boil for 10 minutes. Add chopped parsley
7. Serve soup with a lemon wedge and fresh whole wheat bread or whole grain brown Basmati rice.
8. Enjoy!

2. Carrot and Celery Soup

Great for your skin and eyesight

Serves: 6
Preparation time: 15 minutes
Cooking time: 1 hour 10 minutes

Ingredients

6 carrots
4 small parsley roots
1 celeriac
2 leeks
1 small onion
12 cups of water
3 cloves garlic
2 celery sticks
2 tbsp coconut oil
a dash of pepper

Recipes

1 tsp himalayan salt
1 tbsp black sesame seeds
1/4 cup broccoli sprouts

Instructions:

1. Wash carrots, parsley root and celeriac and cut into cubes.
2. Cut leeks and onions into circles and fry in coconut oil.
3. Add carrots, parsley root and celeriac. Add spices.
4. Place in a pot with water. Bring to boil. Cover and gently simmer for about 1 hour.
5. If you wish: transfer soup to a food processor or blender while adding 1 cup of water. Blend well.
6. Serve soup into individual dishes and sprinkle with black sesame seeds on top.
7. Serve soup with whole grain brown rice with lentils.
8. Enjoy!

3. Stir Fry Tofu, Mushroom Combination and Vegetables

Rich in so many vitamins and minerals and a real boost to your immune system with low fat and calorie content!

Serves: 4
Preparation time: 20 minutes
Cooking time: 10 minutes

Ingredients

1 pack tofu
2 tbs coconut oil
1/2 cup seaweed
1 1/2 onions
1/2 kg (18 oz) fresh green beans

Recipes

4 Shiitake mushrooms
2 forest mushrooms
1 Portobello mushroom
1 tsp chopped ginger
1 tsp curry
1/2 tsp himalayan salt
1/4 cup black sesame seeds
2 garlic cloves
2 tbs soya sauce

Instructions:

1. Soak seaweed in water for 15 minutes
2. Slice tofu into cubes and stir fry in wok with coconut oil and curry until it takes on the color. Place on the side
3. Slice onions and chop garlic, stir fry in remaining oil in wok.
4. Chop the ends off the beans and cut in halves. Add to onion and garlic in the wok for a quick stir fry.
5. Cut mushrooms into 4 parts. Add to wok and stir fry for three more minutes.

Recipes

6. Add to the wok the tofu and seaweed.
7. Sprinkle with sesame seeds
8. Serve soup with round whole grain brown rice.
9. Enjoy!

Recipes

4. Brown Rice and Lentil Stuffed Tomato Cups

An elegant, healthy, satisfying meal - great for special occasions!

Serves: 4
Preparation time: 30 minutes
Cooking time: 1 hour 30 minutes

Ingredients

9 ripe tomatoes
3 tbs coconut oil
13 large onions
1 cup round whole grain (brown) rice
1/4 cup tomato paste
1 cup parsley
1 cup red lentils
1/2 tsp black pepper

Recipes

1/2 tsp himalayan salt
3.5-4 cups of water

Instructions:

1. Arrange tomatoes on chopping board. Cut bases off from tomatoes. Scoop out the seeds and flesh from inside the tomatoes so as to form tomato cups.
2. Chop the flesh from the tomatoes. Chop onions.
3. Heat coconut oil and fry onions over low heat. Add rice and lentils. Stir for 3 minutes. Add chopped tomato flesh and tomato paste. Bring to boil. Reduce heat, cover and allow to simmer for 7 minutes. Remove from heat. Stir in the salt, pepper, and parsley.
4. Preheat oven to 180 °C (360 °F)
5. Spoon mixture into tomato cups. Arrange filled tomatoes in a deep tempered glass baking dish with cover. Pour water into dish. Cover with the top.
6. Bake for 60 minutes

Recipes

7. Remove top and bake for another 30 minutes
8. Baste with pan juice just before serving
9. Serve dish with leafy green salad.
10. Enjoy!

You may exchange the tomatoes for bell peppers, onions or even potatoes!

Recipes

5. Couscous With Chick Pea and Vegetable Soup

Serves: 4
Preparation time: 12 hours
Cooking time: 3 hours

Ingredients

1/2 cup chick peas
7 oz pumpkin
1 courgette
5 carrots
1 parsley root
1 celery root
5 celery sicks
1/4 cabbage
1 leek
2 garlic cloves
1 onion
1/2 cup parsley chopped

1/2 cup coriander chopped
2 tsp curry
2 tsp turmeric
Pinch of Himalayan salt
Pinch of black pepper
8 cups water

For the couscous:
1/2 cup couscous
1 tbs coconut oil
2 cups boiling water
1 tsp turmeric

Instructions:

1. For the soup: Soak the chick peas in water overnight. Wash chickpeas and cover in paper towel to allow to sprout.
2. Place chickpeas in a pot and cover with 8 cups of water. Bring to boil for 10 minutes and reduce heat to simmer for 2 hours.
3. Wash Vegetables and cut to cubes.

4. Place vegetables at the bottom of a pot. Add spices, and chick peas.
5. Bring to boil for 1 minute. Reduce to a simmer for 1 1/2 more hours
6. Add parsley and coriander during the last 10 minutes of cooking
7. For the couscous: Place all ingredients in a bowl and allow to stand for 5 minutes.
8. Fork the couscous until there are no chunks.
9. Place in a fine stainless steel colander above the soup.
10. Steam for 20 minutes.
11. Serve the couscous on the bottom of a serving bowl, cover with soup.
12. Enjoy!

Recipes

6. Vegan Soup Stock

Rich in nutrients and flavor, a must for every vegan or vegetarian soup!

Serves: 6-8
Preparation time: 15 minutes
Cooking time: 45 minutes

Ingredients

1 large carrot
1 onion
3 stalks celery,
2 leeks
3 garlic cloves
1 parsley stem and 2 parsley leaves,
3 bay leaves

Recipes

1 tsp fennel seeds
1 tsp coriander seeds
1 8-inch (20 cm) sheet of Kombu seaweed
2 cups of dried oyster, shiitake, wood ear and porcini mushrooms

Instructions:

1. Place all of the ingredients together in a large pot.
2. Cover and bring to boil.
3. Reduce heat and allow to simmer for 45 minutes or until all vegetables are soft, stirring occasionally.
4. Strain soup through a fine strainer.
5. Allow stock to cool for 1 hour at room temperature.
6. Use for soup immediately or refrigerate and use throughout the week for other dishes.
7. Enjoy!

Recipes

7. Vegan Bean Soup

Serves: 6-8
Preparation time: 12 hours
Cooking time: 30 minutes

Ingredients

1 Onion
2 tbs coconut oil
2 cups of vegan stock (see recipe)
2 cups beans soaked overnight
1/2 cup tomato paste
3 garlic cloves
1/4 cup parsley
1 tbsp peppercorns
1/2 tsp black pepper
1/2 tsp himalayan salt
4 cups of water

Instructions:

1. Soak the beans for a day refreshing the water after 12 hours.
2. Chop the flesh from the tomatoes. Chop onions.
3. Heat coconut oil and fry onions over low heat in a large pot. Stir for 3 minutes. Add vegan soup stock, beans, tomato paste, garlic, pepper, salt and parsley. Add 2 cups of water.
4. Bring to boil. Reduce heat, and cook for 20 minutes.
5. Serve dish with whole wheat pita bread.
6. Enjoy!

8. Brown Lentil Stew

Great smell and great taste! Rich in insoluble fiber which helps balance blood sugar levels by providing a slow and steady energy source!

Serves: 6-8
Preparation time: 20 minutes
Cooking time: 1 hour 30 minutes

Ingredients

1 cup brown lentils
2 tbs whole grain cooked barley or rice (see recipe # 50)
1/2 cup soaked wood ear mushrooms
1 onion
1/4 cup chopped parsley
1 tbsp peppercorns
1/2 tsp all spice

Recipes

1/2 tsp cumin
1/2 tsp himalayan salt
6 cups of water

Instructions:

1. Soak lentils and mushrooms for 15 minutes, wash and rinse.
2. Place in a pot with 6 cups water. Bring to boil
3. Cover and simmer for 1 hour and 20 minutes.
4. Transfer soup to a blender, add 1 cup water and blend.
5. Return the mixture to the pot, add spices, salt .
6. Chop onion and fry in coconut oil. Add to lentil mixture. Bring to second boil for 10 minutes.
7. Add parsley to stew.
8. Serve dish with whole grain cooked barley or rice.
9. Enjoy!

9. Special Green Lentils with Chard or Bok Choy

A nutritious soup rich in protein, vitamins A, C, and K, as well as magnesium, potassium, and iron with a special flavour!

Serves: 6-8
Preparation time: 15 minutes
Cooking time: 1 hour 10 minutes

Ingredients

1 cup green lentils
1/2 kg (16 oz) Swiss chard or Pak choy, chopped
3 potatoes
2 garlic cloves
1/2 cup finely chopped coriander
1/4 cup squeezed lemon juice
4 cups water

Recipes

2 small onions
1 stalk celery
1/4 cup chopped parsley
1 tbsp peppercorns
1/2 tsp cumin
1/2 tsp himalayan salt

Instructions:

1. Soak lentils for 20 minutes, wash and rinse.
2. Place in a pot with water. Bring to boil
3. Cover and simmer for 25 minutes.
4. Add green leaves (Swiss chard or Bok choy), celery and diced potatoes. Continue to cook for 15 minutes
5. Chop onion and fry with garlic and cumin in coconut oil for a minute. Add to lentil mixture along with lemon juice. Bring to second boil and cook for 10 more minutes.
6. Serve dish with brown Basmati rice.
7. Enjoy!

10. Mediterranean Fava Bean Dish

A nutritious dish with a special surprising flavour!

Serves: 6
Preparation time: 24 hours
Cooking time: 1 hour 30 minutes

Ingredients

1 1/2 cups fava beans
1/2 cup squeezed lemon juice
3 garlic cloves
1/2 cup finely chopped coriander
3 cups water
1/4 cup finely chopped parsley
1/2 tsp cumin

Recipes

Instructions:

1. Soak fava beans for 24 hours, replacing the water after 12 hours.
2. Place fresh fava beans in a heat proof sieve and place sieve with beans in a pot with water. Bring to boil for 1 minute. Remove sieve from water, and place beans in a bowl with ice. This will help you discard tough skins.
3. Place peeled fava beans in a pot with water. Bring to boil and lower the heat. Simmer for 1 hour and 30 minutes. Allow to cool.
4. Mix garlic, lemon juice, cumin, cayenne pepper, chopped parsley and a table spoon of olive oil.
5. Lightly mash cooked fava beans.
6. Serve with fresh onion, tomato and a whole grain pita bread.
7. Enjoy!

11. Home-made Hummus

A healthy, satisfying, tasty and nutritious dish!

Serves: 6-8
Preparation time: 24 hours
Cooking time: 1 hour 30 minutes

Ingredients

1 1/2 cups fava beans
1/2 cup squeezed lemon juice
3 garlic cloves
1/2 cup finely chopped coriander
3 cups water
1/4 cup finely chopped parsley
1/2 tsp cumin

Instructions:

1. Soak chick beans for 24 hours, replacing the water after 12 hours.
2. Place chick peas in a pot with water. Bring to boil for 1 minute lower the heat. Simmer for 1 hour and 30 minutes. Allow to cool.
3. Once soft, drain warm chickpeas. Set 2 tsp of whole cooked chick peas aside to decorate dish.
4. Blend chick peas with whole seed sesame paste, lemon juice, garlic and salt.
5. Place in individual bowls garnish with red pepper, a parsley twig and whole chick peas.
6. Serve with fresh onion and a whole grain pita.
7. Enjoy!

Recipes

12. Red Lentil Soup

Serves: 4
Preparation time: 2 minutes
Cooking time: 30 minutes

Ingredients

1 1/2 cups red lentils
3 bay leaves
1 tsp turmeric
1 tsp cumin
1/2 tsp cayenne pepper
1/2 squeezed lemon juice
2 garlic cloves
1/2 cup finely chopped coriander
6 cups vegan soup stock - (see recipe # 6)
1/4 cup finely chopped parsley
2 tbs coconut oil or ghee
2 tsp mustard seeds
Himalayan salt and a dash of pepper

Instructions:

1. Rinse lentils in a sieve under running water.
2. Place in a pot with vegan stock, turmeric, Cayenne, cumin and bay leaves.
3. Bring to boil and then reduce the heat and allow to simmer until the lentils are very soft (ca 25 minutes).
4. Remove bay leaves.
5. Mash the lentils with a ladle).
6. Sauté the onion, garlic and mustard seeds for 2 minutes in the coconut oil and add to the soup.
7. Let simmer for another 5 minutes.
8. Add salt, pepper and squeezed lemon.
9. Serve with fresh onion and a whole grain pita.
10. Enjoy!

13. Luscious Tomato Sauce with Peas and Spinach

A healthy, satisfying, tasty and nutritious dish!

Serves: 4
Preparation time: 20 minutes
Cooking time: 2 hours 20 minutes

Ingredients

10 small tomatoes
4 spinach leaves
1/2 cup peas
2 stalks celery
1 onion
2 carrots
4 garlic cloves

1/4 cup tomato paste
2 tbs olive oil
1 tbs coconut oil
1/4 cup chopped fresh basil
1/4 cup red wine
1 bay leaf
Himalayan salt and a dash of pepper

Instructions:

1. Bring a pot of water to a boil. Place whole tomatoes in boiling water until skin starts to peel. Since under cold water and remove the peels.
2. Chop 8 tomatoes and keep their seeds. Place the 8 in a blender and blend. Chop the two remaining tomatoes and set aside.
3. Chop onion and carrot. Mince garlic. Sauté all three in pot with oil for 2 minutes.
4. Pour into the pot pureed tomatoes. Stir in chopped tomato, basil and wine. Place bay leaf and whole celery stalks in pot. Bring to a boil, then reduce heat.
5. Simmer 2 hours.

Recipes

6. Stir in tomato paste and simmer for another 1 1/2 hours. Add spinach and peas. Simmer for 30 minutes longer. Discard bay leaf and celery.
7. Serve with whole durum wheat pasta.
8. Enjoy!

This sauce can be frozen in separate portions to be used when needed.

Recipes

14. Sprouted Black Lentil Soup

A perfectly balanced vegan meal!

Serves: 4
Preparation time: 12 hours
Cooking time: 2 hours

Ingredients

2 cups black lentils
1 tomato
1 tbs coconut oil
1 tbs fresh ginger
6 garlic cloves
3 cups water
2 tsp curry powder
1 tsp cumin
1 tsp black pepper

enough water to cover all ingredients

Instructions:

1. Soak black lentils for 12 hours. Drain and wash the lentils
2. Wrap in a paper towel and place on a plate in a dark corner for 12 hours and allow to sprout (wash every few hours)
3. Grind the tomato and ginger, and mince the garlic. Place them in a stock pot with the cumin, curry powder, black pepper and oil. Sauté for 2 minutes.
4. Add the lentils and water to the pot and bring to boil for 1 minute.
5. Lower the heat. Simmer for 2 hours.
6. For those who prefer a smoother soup, you can place the soup in the blender.
7. Serve with a mixture of long grain brown and wild rice or accompany with mashed potatoes.
8. Enjoy!

15. Mediterranean Salad

A Nutritious compliment to any meal!

Serves: 4
Preparation time: 15 minutes

Ingredients

2 cucumbers
3 tomato
1 red pepper
4 radishes
1/5 purple cabbage
2 tbs chopped parsley
1 tbs natural balsamic vinegar
1 tsp Himalayan salt
1/4 tsp ground pepper

Instructions:

1. Wash and dry all vegetables
2. You may wish to peel the cucumbers
3. Remove seeds and stem of pepper
4. Dice/cut all vegetables or use a hand powered salad chopper making sure you chop each vegetable separately.
5. Place in a bowl
6. Sprinkle with natural balsamic vinegar.
7. Add salt and pepper. Toss salad.
8. Serve with tahini spread. See recipe # 16
9. Enjoy!

16. Tahini Spread

Another Nutritious compliment to any meal!

Serves: 4-6
Preparation time: 15 minutes

Ingredients

1 1/2 cups whole grain sprouted sesame seed paste
1 cup water
1/2 cup fresh lemon juice
2 cloves garlic
1/2 tsp paprika
1 tsp ground pepper
1 parsley twig
1/2 tsp Himalayan salt

Instructions:

1. Pour sesame seed paste into a deep bowl and add the water slowly stirring the mixture consistently with a fork.
2. Add lemon juice and keep stirring until the paste become smooth and creamy.
3. Add salt, garlic, paprika, and pepper. Keep stirring.
4. Decorate with some paprika and chopped parsley.
5. Serve as a salad dressing or as a vegetable dip.
6. Enjoy!

17. Mung Beans and Spinach Stew

A colourful and hearty vegan meal!

Serves: 4-6
Preparation time: 12 hours
Cooking time: 1 hour 15 minutes

Ingredients

1 1/2 cups dried mung beans
3 onions
2 tbs coconut oil
2 tbs freshly minced ginger
1 tsp paprika
1 tsp black pepper
5 garlic cloves
14 oz coconut milk

Recipes

1 tbs soy sauce
2 cups chopped spinach leaves
1/2 tsp Himalayan salt

Instructions:

1. Soak mung beans in water for 12 hours. Drain.
2. Place beans in a pot, cover with water and bring to boil for 2 minutes.
3. Reduce heat and simmer for 1 hour. Drain and rinse.
4. In a wok or large pan, sauté onions in the coconut oil with salt.
5. Add ginger, paprika, black pepper, and garlic. Simmer on low heat for 2 minutes.
6. Add the coconut milk and simmer for 5 more minutes.
7. Add the mung beans to onion and spice mix.
8. Add soy sauce and spinach and cook for 10 minutes
9. Serve with red indian whole grain rice.
10. Enjoy!

18. Brown Rice Risotto With Asparagus

Serves: 4
Preparation time: 15 minutes
Cooking time: 1 hour 10 minutes

Ingredients

1 cup whole grain round risotto rice
1 onion
1 tbs coconut oil
5 cloves of garlic
10 asparagus spears
1 cup fresh or dried mushrooms
1 tsp dried thyme
1/2 cup dry white wine
6 cups vegan stock, see recipe # 6
2 cups Swiss chard
1 tbs freshly squeezed lemon juice
1/2 tsp Himalayan salt
1 oz sliced almonds

Instructions:

1. Chop onion, mince garlic and cut head of asparagus.
2. Heat pot, add onion, garlic, and asparagus to coconut oil and sauté for 5 minutes.
3. Add mushrooms, thyme, salt, and dry white wine, and cook for 5 minutes.
4. Add rice to mixture and cook for 3 minutes.
5. Add vegetable stock 1/2 cup every 5-6 minutes, stirring well.
6. After adding the stock liquid, add the Swiss chard and lemon juice and stir for 5 minutes. Cook for 50 minutes.
7. Lightly toast sliced almonds and sprinkle on top of risotto before serving.
8. Serve and Enjoy!

19. Whole Wheat Pasta with Cauliflower and Nut Sauce

A creamy, tasty cholesterol free super tasty pasta sauce!

Serves: 4-6
Preparation time: 20 minutes
Cooking time: 50 minutes

Ingredients

2 cups whole grain pasta of your choice
Cauliflower sauce:
1 cauliflower head
1 tbs coconut oil
4 cloves of garlic
1 spring onion
1/2 cup whole grain sesame paste
1 tbs ground cumin

1 tsp paprika
1/2 tsp cayenne pepper
2 tbs whole grain flour of your choice
1 1/2 cups non sweetened almond milk
1 tsp Himalayan salt

Pasta Topping

1 cup walnuts
1 tsp freshly squeezed lemon juice
1/2 tsp ground pepper
1 tsp Himalayan salt
1 cup whole wheat bread crumbs
1 tbs coconut oil

Instructions:

1. Preheat oven to 350 degrees F (180 degrees C)
2. Cook pasta according to instructions on package. Drain and return to pot.
3. Cauliflower sauce: Place cauliflower florets in pot and cover with water

4. Bring to boil and cook for 10 minutes until soft. Drain
5. In a pan heat oil, garlic and spring onion. Sauté for 3 minutes.
6. Add the sesame paste, cumin, paprika, cayenne pepper, salt and flour. Stir until it thickens.
7. Add almond milk slowly and keep stirring.
8. Place cauliflower florets with sesame seed mixture into a blender and blend until smooth. Remove from blender and place on the side
9. Topping: Blend the nuts, lemon, pepper and salt in a food processor or coffee grinder. Add the bread crumbs and a tbs of oil and mix together.
10. Place on a baking tray lightly coated with oil and place in the preheated oven.
11. Stir sauce into the pasta pot, add more water if needed. Then pour mixture into baking tray and place in oven. Sprinkle with breadcrumb topping and bake for 15 minutes.
12. Serve and Enjoy!

Recipes

Recipes

20. Quinoa, Red Lentil and Wheat Groat Mix

Serves: 4-6
Preparation time: 12 hours
Cooking time: 35 minutes

Ingredients

1/2 cup Quinoa
!/2 cup red lentils
1/2 cup wheat groats
1 onion
2 garlic cloves
2 tbs coconut oil
1/4 lemon grind
1/4 tsp spicy paprika
Pinch of Himalayan salt
Pinch black pepper

Instructions:

1. Soak wheat groats overnight. Drain and rinse.
2. Chop onion. In a pot, heat coconut oil, add chopped onion and sauté for 3 minutes. Add garlic and sauté for 1 more minute.
3. Add all other ingredients to pot. Stir.
4. Add 3 cups of water. Cover and bring to boil for 3 minutes
5. Reduce heat and simmer for 30 minutes stirring occasionally.
6. Sprinkle on top some garlic pepper seasoning if desired and serve.
7. Enjoy!

21. Buckwheat Noodles with Snow Peas and Asparagus

Serves: 4
Preparation time: 15 minutes
Cooking time: 25 minutes

Ingredients

1 pack buckwheat (Udon) noodles
1 onion
8 oz snow peas
8 oz asparagus
4 oz chopped mushrooms
2 tbs sesame seed oil
3 cloves garlic
6 tbs soy sauce or Tamari
1 tbs grated ginger
Pinch of Himalayan salt
Pinch black pepper
1 tbs sesame seeds

Instructions:

1. Cook noodles according to package instructions. Rinse in water to remove stickiness.
2. Cut asparagus into pieces same size as snow peas.
3. Heat sesame oil in a walk or large pan. Add onion, snow peas, asparagus, mushrooms, and ginger.
4. Stir fry 7-10 minutes.
5. Add soy sauce, sesame seeds and the noodles.
6. Toss and cook for 5 more minutes.
7. Serve and enjoy!

22. Whole wheat Rice Noodles with Bean Sprouts and Shelled Edamame

Serves: 4
Preparation time: 10 minutes
Cooking time: 25 minutes

Ingredients

1 pack wholewheat rice noodles
8 oz mushrooms sliced
8 oz cut spring onion
5 oz bean sprouts
5 oz shelled edamame
1 oz fresh ginger, minced
2 garlic cloves, minced
1/3 cup water
1/3 cup soy sauce or Tamari
1/3 cup rice wine vinegar
Pinch of Himalayan salt

Recipes

Instructions:

1. Cook noodles according to package instructions. Rinse in water to remove stickiness.
2. Heat sesame oil in a wok or large frying pan.
3. Add spring onion, mushrooms, bean sprouts, shelled edamame, ginger, garlic and salt.
4. Stir fry for 7 minutes
5. Stir in the water, soy sauce and vinegar. Bring to a boil.
6. Add the noodles.
7. Toss and cook for 5 more minutes.
8. Serve and enjoy!

Recipes

23. Tofu and Vegetable Bake

Serves: 4
Preparation time: 20 minutes
Cooking time: 1 hour 10 minutes

Ingredients

20 oz extra firm organic tofu, drained and washed
3 tbs coconut oil
1/2 cup chopped parsley
8 oz carrot coins
8 oz broccoli florets
8 oz green peas
4 garlic cloves minced
1/4 cup soy or tamari sauce.
 pack wholewheat rice noodles
Pinch of Himalayan salt
Pinch of black pepper

Instructions:

1. Preheat oven to 350 degrees F (180 degrees C)
2. In a bowl, crumble the tofu to look like shredded cheese.
3. Add 2 tbs coconut oil, parsley salt and pepper. Mix
4. Spread half of the tofu mixture on a baking dish (23X33 cm)
5. In another mixing bowl toss together all vegetables with minced garlic, soy sauce, 1 tbs coconut oil, salt and pepper to taste.
6. Spread vegetables on the tofu in the baking dish.
7. Sprinkle remaining tofu on top of the vegetables.
8. Bake for 35 minutes until top begins to brown and carrots are tender.
9. Serve and enjoy!

24. Cannellini Beans With Olives

Serves: 4
Preparation time: 20 minutes
Cooking time: 50 minutes

Ingredients

15 oz fresh cannellini beans (no need to used canned versions, fresh ones are easy to prepare.
2 red onions
2 tbs coconut oil
4 garlic cloves
1/2 cup green or black olives
Tomato paste
2 tsp dried oregano
1/2 cup water
Pinch of Himalayan salt
Pinch of black pepper

Instructions:

1. No soaking required. Place water in a pot to cover the beans. Bring beans to boil for 10 minutes.
2. Reduce to medium heat and cook for about 20 to 30 minutes or until the beans are soft. Drain and rinse.
3. In a pan, heat oil and sauté onion and garlic.
4. Add the beans, olives, tomato paste, water, salt and pepper
5. Bring to boil, lower heat and simmer for 20 minutes. Stir occasionally.
6. Serve and enjoy!

25. Vegan Sushi With Whole Grain Rice

Serves: 4
Preparation time: 12 hours
Cooking time: 45 minutes

Ingredients

2 cups whole grain round rice
4 sheets of sushi nori paper
1 tbs sesame oil
1 tsp black sesame seeds
1 tbs mustard
2 spring onions cut into strips
1 cucumber cut into sticks
1 carrots cut into sticks
1 avocado cut into sticks
1 handful sunflower seed sprouts
1 cup tofu marinated in soy sauce and steamed in the oven for 10 minutes
For serving: Wasabi, ginger slices and soy sauce.

Recipes

Instructions:

1. The rice: Soak the rice overnight. Drain and wash.
2. Place the rice in a pot, with 5 cups of water
3. Bring to boil for 5 minutes and reduce heat to a simmer for 40 minutes when all water is absorbed.
4. Remove from heat. Add sesame oil and sesame seeds to the rice and allow to stand.
5. The sushi: On a sushi rolling mat place a nori sheet with the rough side up
6. Spread the rice on the nori sheet evenly.
7. Place the vegetables and sprouts on the rice.
8. Scatter the sunflower seeds on the vegetables
9. Roll the sushi and pat it. Remove the rolling mat.
10. Slice the roll into 4 or 6 pieces
11. Serve with wasabi sauce, ginger slices and soy sauce.
12. Enjoy!

26. Aubergine Salad

Serves: 4-6
Preparation time: 12 hours
Cooking time: 45 minutes

Ingredients

2 eggplants
1/4 cup lemon juice
1 tomato
1 bell pepper
1/4 cup parsley
2 spring onions
1 tsp garlic powder
Pinch of Himalayan salt
Pinch of black pepper
3 tbs whole sesame seed paste

Recipes

Instructions:

1. Preheat the oven to 400 degree F (200 degrees C)
2. Rinse and pat dry aubergines. Do not peel.
3. Place on a backing dish in the oven for 40 minutes, turning occasionally.
4. Remove from oven and place whole aubergine under running cold water.
5. Scoop out the flesh and immediately pour freshly squeezed lemon juice over it.
6. Mash the flesh with a fork.
7. Add chopped onion, pepper, spring onion, sesame seed paste and all seasonings. Mix.
8. Serve with Whole grain Pita bread.
9. Enjoy!

27. Broad Beans with Artichokes

Serves: 4-6
Preparation time: 12 hours
Cooking time: 1 hour 15 minutes

Ingredients

1 cup broad beans (fresh or frozen)
2 1/2 cups water
2 onions
2 tbs dill
2 tbs coconut oil
2 tbs lemon juice
1 cup frozen peas
2 cups frozen artichoke bottoms (or drained artichoke hearts from a jar)
4 spring onions, chopped
Pinch of Himalayan salt
Pinch of black pepper

Instructions:

1. Soak broad beans in water for 12 hours. Drain and rinse.
2. Place broad beans in a pot and cover with water. Cover pot. Bring to boil for 2 minutes. Rinse under cold water and peel beans.
3. Return to pot and add 2 1/2 cups of water. Bring to boil.
4. Reduce heat and simmer for 50 minutes until broad beans are soft.
5. Slice onions into rings. Chop dill.
6. Heat oil in large pan. Add onions. Sauté for 5 minutes.
7. Add broad beans, water and lemon juice to pan. Cover and bring to boil for 1 minute.
8. Reduce heat and simmer for 5 minutes.
9. Add frozen peas, artichokes and seasoning.
10. Simmer mixture (covered) for 5 minutes until peas are tender.
11. Remove from heat. Add spring onions, salt and pepper.
12. Garnish with dill.

Recipes

13. Serve on mashed potatoes.
14. Enjoy!

Recipes

28. White Beans with Zucchini

Serves: 4-6
Preparation time: 12 hours
Cooking time: 55 minutes

Ingredients

1 cup white beans (fresh or frozen)
3 cups water
2 small pickling onions
1 tbs coconut oil
2 cloves garlic, minced
4 tomatoes
1 tbs lemon juice
1 1/2 cups tomato juice
2 tbs red wine
18 oz zucchini
1 tbs fresh ground oregano
Pinch of Himalayan salt

Pinch of black pepper
4 rocket leaves
4 cherry tomatoes

Instructions:

1. Soak beans in water overnight. Drain and rinse.
2. Heat oil in a pan. Add onions and garlic. Sauté for 5 minutes.
3. Add tomatoes, beans, tomato juice, lemon juice and wine.
4. Simmer covered for 40 minutes.
5. Add zucchini and simmer for another 10 minuets.
6. Stir in oregano, and pepper.
7. Serve on brown rice.
8. Garnish with rocket leaves and sliced cherry tomatoes
9. Enjoy!

29. Green Beans and New Potatoes

Serves: 4
Preparation time: 15 minutes
Cooking time: 25 minutes

Ingredients

18 oz baby new potatoes
9 oz green beans
3 kale leaves
2 tbs olive oil
2 red chillies
1 clove garlic
1/4 cup fresh coriander
1 tbs red wine vinegar
1/2 tsp caraway seeds
Pinch of Himalayan salt
Pinch of black pepper

Instructions:

1. Cut potatoes into four.
2. Place potatoes in large pan. Cover with water. Bring to boil for 1 minute.
3. Simmer for 20 minutes. Remove from heat.
4. Blanch beans and kale in boiling water for 2 minutes. Drain and set aside.
5. In a bowl mix together olive oil, chillies, garlic, coriander, red wine vinegar and caraway seeds.
6. Place all ingredients in a bowl and mix together 5 minutes before serving.
7. Garnish with parsley.
8. Enjoy!

30. Black Beans and Pasta

Serves: 4
Preparation time: 15 minutes
Cooking time: 2 hours

Ingredients

2 cups black beans
10 oz pasta of your choice
2 tbs coconut oil
1 onion
1 red onion
1/2 cup spinach
6 tomatoes, chopped
3 cloves garlic, minced
9 cups water
2 bay leaves
1 tbs paprika
1 tbs cumin
1 tbs coriander
Pinch of Himalayan salt
1 tbs black pepper

Instructions:

1. Soak beans overnight.
2. Drain and rinse.
3. In a large pot, heat oil. Add onions and garlic. Sauté for 5-10 minutes
4. Add water, bay leaves, paprika, black pepper, cumin, coriander, beans, spinach, tomatoes with their juice. Stir
5. Bring to boil for 1 minute and reduce heat to a simmer for 1 1/2-2 hours, stirring occasionally.
6. Remove bay leaves.
7. Cook pasta according to package instructions. Drain and rinse.
8. Add pasta to bean soup and mix.
9. Garnish with parsley and avocado.
10. Enjoy!

31. Cannellini, Aubergine and Sweet Potato Ragout

Serves: 4
Preparation time: 20 minutes
Cooking time: 2 hours

Ingredients

1 cup cannellini beans
1 aubergine
2 tbs coconut oil
4 sweet potatoes
2 onions
2 cloves garlic, minced
2 tbs ginger, grated
1 tbs cumin
1/4 tsp black pepper
6 tomatoes
Pinch of Himalayan salt
1 spring onions cut for garnish

Instructions:

1. Preheat oven to 400 degrees F (200 degree C)
2. Place aubergine in a baking dish.
3. Roast aubergine in oven for 30-40 minutes. Remove from oven and place to cool. When cooled slit aubergine open and cut out cubes of flesh.
4. Place beans in a pot and cover with water. Bring beans to boil for 10 minutes. Reduce to medium heat and cook for about 20 to 30 minutes or until the beans are soft. Drain and rinse.
5. In a pan, heat oil and sauté onion and garlic ginger and potatoes for 5 minutes.
6. Stir in cumin, salt and pepper.
7. Add aubergine cubes and the tomatoes and their juice. Bring to boil for 1 minute.
8. Reduce heat and simmer for 20 minutes.
9. Add the beans. Cover and simmer for 10 more minutes.
10. Garnish with spring onion.
11. Serve and enjoy!

32. White Wine Roasted Potatoes, Peas and Kale

Serves: 4
Preparation time: 10 minutes
Cooking time: 50 minutes

Ingredients

1 1/4 pound baby potatoes
1 red onion
6 leaves kale
2/3 cup frozen peas
1/4 cup dry white wine
1 tbs white wine vinegar
2 tbs Dijon mustard
2 cloves garlic
Pinch of Himalayan salt
1 spring onions cut for garnish

Instructions:

1. Preheat oven to 400 degrees F (200 degree C)
2. Cut kale, chop onions and halve potatoes.
3. Combine all seasonings, garlic, mustard, wine and vinegar in a bowl. Add potatoes, kale and onion.
4. Place in a deep baking dish with cover.
5. Place in oven covered for 30 minutes. Remove cover, stir potatoes, add peas and kale. Bake for 20 more minutes.
6. Serve and enjoy!

33. Potatoes with Asparagus Au Gratin

Serves: 4
Preparation time: 15 minutes
Cooking time: 1 hour 15 minutes

Ingredients

1 3/4 pound potatoes
12 oz tofu, extra firm
2 tbs sesame seed oil
1/2 cup soy or rice creamer
2 tbs miso soup powder
1 tbs garlic powder
1 tbs paprika
1/2 tsp turmeric
7 oz asparagus spears
1 red onion
Pinch of Himalayan salt
1 spring onions cut for garnish

Instructions:

1. Preheat oven to 350 degrees F (180 degree C)
2. Slice potatoes and rinse.
3. In a blender, add tofu, oil, creamer, miso, garlic powder, paprika, onion, turmeric, salt and pepper. Blend until smooth.
4. In a bowl, combine potatoes and sauce from blender. Spread mixture on a deep baking dish with lid (8 X 8-inch, 20 X 20-cm).
5. Bake, covered for 45 minutes. Remove lid, add asparagus and bake for an additional 30 minutes.
6. Remove from heat for 10 minutes before serving.
7. Serve and enjoy!

34. Mashed Potatoes with Spinach Served with Corn on the Cob

Serves: 4
Preparation time: 15 minutes
Cooking time: 60 minutes

Ingredients

2 1/2 pound potatoes
4 ears fresh corn on the cob
1 pound spinach fresh or frozen
3 tbs mustard
2 tbs coconut oil
Pinch pepper to taste
Pinch of Himalayan salt

Instructions:

1. Cut potatoes (leaving the peel)
2. Boil in salted water until tender (approximately 40 minutes)
3. Cut spinach into small pieces and place in a pot. (if you use frozen spinach, prepare according to instructions), add a dash of lemon juice and cook for 7 minutes.
4. Clean corn and place in a pot. Cover with water and bring to boil for 5 minutes. Reduce heat and simmer for 10 more minutes. Remove from heat and drain water.
5. Drain potatoes and return to pot. Add spinach, oil, salt, pepper and mustard to potatoes. Mash all together.
6. Serve with corn on the cob.
7. Enjoy!

35. Red Bean Jambalaya

Serves: 4
Preparation time: 12 hours
Cooking time: 3 hours

Ingredients

2 cups red beans
1 cup brown long grain rice
1/2 cup wild rice
2 tbs coconut oil
1 green or orange bell pepper
2 onions
3 stalks celery
3 cups vegan stock - see recipe # 6)
1/4 cup soy sauce
1 cup water
Pinch pepper to taste
Pinch of Himalayan salt

Recipes

Instructions:

1. Soak red beans in water for 12 hours. Drain and rinse.
2. Soak both types of rice together for 2 hours. Drain and rinse.
3. Place beans in a pot and cover with water. Cover pot. Bring to boil for 2 minutes. Reduce heat and simmer for 2 hours until beans are soft.
4. Chop pepper, onions and celery.
5. In a pan, heat oil over medium heat. Add pepper, onions and celery. Cover and cook for 15 minutes.
6. Add stock and soy sauce. Bring to boil for 1 minute and reduce heat to a simmer for 20 minutes, covered.
7. Add rice. Cover and bring to boil. Reduce heat to a simmer for 30 minutes.
8. Add beans, stir for 5 minutes.
9. Serve and enjoy!

Recipes

36. Tri Colored Rice Paella

Serves: 4
Preparation time: 1 hour
Cooking time: 50 minutes

Ingredients

2 1/2 cups brown Basmati rice
2 leeks
4 celery stalks
4 garlic cloves
1 red bell pepper
1 tomato
1/2 cup tofu
10 shiitake mushrooms
4 forest mushrooms
2 tbs coconut oil
2 tbs soya sauce
1/2 tsp curry powder
2 tbs ginger
1/2 tsp chilli powder

3 cups vegan stock (see recipe # 6)
1 cup coriander
Pinch pepper to taste
Pinch of Himalayan salt

Instructions:

1. Cube tofu and mushrooms. Place in a bowl. Marinate with soy sauce, ginger, and curry powder for 1 hour
2. Place rice in a bowl. Cover with water and soak for 1 hour. Drain and rinse.
3. Preheat oven to 350 degree F (180 degrees C).
4. In an oven proof pan with lid, heat oil and sauté onion, leek and garlic until golden.
5. Add the rice, vegetables and seasonings. Stir.
6. Add vegan stock and bring to boil. Reduce heat and simmer for 10 minutes.
7. Remove from heat and place in oven, covered, for 30 minutes.
8. Remove cover, stir, add tofu cubes and mushrooms. Bake for 10 more minutes.
9. Serve and enjoy!

37. Quinoa, Mexican Style

Serves: 4
Preparation time: 12 hours
Cooking time: 2 hours

Ingredients

2 cups tri color quinoa (or normal quinoa)
4 corn stalks
2 cups black beans
6 tomatoes
2 tbs olive oil
1 tbs lemon juice
1/2 tsp cumin
1 tsp garlic powder
1 tsp chilli flakes
Pinch pepper to taste
Pinch of Himalayan salt
1 red onion diced
1 spring onion chopped

Recipes

Instructions:

1. Soak red beans in water for 12 hours. Drain and rinse.
2. Place beans in a pot and cover with 5 cups water. Cover pot. Bring to boil for 2 minutes. Reduce heat and simmer for 2 hours until beans are soft.
3. Clean corn and place in a pot. Cover with water and bring to boil for 5 minutes. Reduce heat and simmer for 15 more minutes. Remove from heat and drain water. Cut off corn kernels from the cob using a sharp knife and set aside.
4. In pot bring 4 cups water to boil. Add quinoa and bring to boil. Reduce heat and simmer for 12 minutes.
5. Remove from heat and fluff quinoa with a fork. Allow to cool.
6. Mix all ingredients except quinoa in a pot. When quinoa cools add it to the pot. Mix.
7. Garnish with onions.
8. Serve and enjoy!

38. Spaghetti and Tofu Sauce

Serves: 4
Preparation time: 15 minutes
Cooking time: 1 hour 10 minutes

Ingredients

1 Pack wholewheat spelt penne pasta
1 cup tofu, cubed
2 tbs coconut oil
1 onion
2 cloves garlic
1 stalk celery
1 carrot
10 tomatoes
6 kale leaves
2 bay leaves
Pinch pepper to taste
Pinch of Himalayan salt

Recipes

Instructions:

1. Prepare penne according to package instructions.
2. In a pot, heat oil over medium heat. Add onion and garlic and sauté for 2 minutes.
3. Add celery, carrots, tofu, kale leaves, salt and pepper.
4. Sauté for 5 minutes. Add tomatoes and bay leaves. Simmer covered on low heat for 1 hour or until thick.
5. Remove from heat and remove bay leaves.
6. Place sauce into blender. Blend until right consistency for you.
7. Place back in pan. Add penne pasta. Heat for 10 minutes or until well mixed and heated.
8. Serve and enjoy!

39. Penne with Pine Kernel Cream Sauce

Serves: 4
Preparation time: 20 minutes
Cooking time: 20 minutes

Ingredients

1 Pack wholewheat spelt spaghetti
10 oz cherry tomatoes, halved
1/2 cup pine kernels
1 tbs coconut oil
2 onions
6 cloves garlic
2 tbs any bean flour
2 cups almond milk (Blue VitaRiz or unsweetened Almond Breeze)
Pinch of Himalayan salt

Instructions:

1. Prepare spaghetti according to package instructions. Drain, cover and set aside.
2. Preheat oven to 400 degrees F (200 degree C).
3. Place in a small pyrex the pine kernels. Allow to roast for 10 minutes. Remove from heat and set aside.
4. Place halved cherry tomatoes on a separate baking dish in oven. Allow to roast for 15 minutes. Remove from heat and set aside.
5. In a large pan add the coconut oil, sauté onions and garlic for 3-4 minutes. Add a pinch of salt and black pepper and stir.
6. Add flour and using a hand whisk, mix. Slowly add the almond milk a little at a time.
7. Add a pinch of salt and black pepper, bring to a simmer and cook for 5 minutes, until thick.
8. Transfer sauce to a blender and blend until smooth.
9. Place back in pan and simmer until thick.
10. Add pasta, pine kernels and roasted tomatoes and stir. Remove from heat. Serve and enjoy!

40. Spaghetti and "Meat" Balls

Serves: 4
Preparation time: 20 minutes
Cooking time: 1 hour 10 minutes

Ingredients

1 Pack wholewheat spelt spaghetti
2 cups lentils
2 tbs coconut oil
1 red onion
1 zucchini
1 carrot
2 stalks celery
2 tbs parsley, chopped
2 tbs flax seeds
1 can organic chopped tomatoes

5 garlic cloves, sliced
1 pinch chilli flakes
1 fresh basil sprig
Pinch of Himalayan salt
1 tbs sugar free balsamic vinegar
1 tbs soy sauce
1 tsp paprika
1 tsp garlic powder
1 cup whole wheat bread crumbs or any gluten free crumbs
1 tbs chopped fresh parsley

Instructions:

1. Prepare spaghetti according to package instructions. Drain, cover and set aside.
2. Rince and drain lentils.
3. In a pot, bring 4 cups of water to a boil. Add the lentils and return to a boil. Lower the heat, cover and allow to simmer for 20 minutes. Let cool.
4. Heat 1 tbs oil in a pan. Add onions and sauté them for 4 minutes.

5. Add the carrots, celery, garlic, salt and pepper. Sauté about 5 minutes until tender. Allow to cool.
6. Preheat oven to 400 degree F (200 degree C)
7. In the meantime prepare the flax seed gel: Place the flax seeds in a bowl. Cover with a few tbs warm water in a bowl. Mix and let stand for 10 minutes until it becomes a gel.
8. Prepare the marinara sauce: Pour canned tomatoes into a large bowl and crush with your hands. Add 1 cup water into can, slosh around and add to the bowl. In a large pan, heat 1 tbs coconut oil. When it is hot, add garlic. Sauté for 1 minute.
9. Add the tomato and water mixture, add chilli, basil sprig and salt. Stir and simmer while preparing the rest of the recipe.
10. Place the cooled lentils and vegetables in a blender. Add parsley, spices and sauces and blend until smooth.
11. Slowly add flax seed gel to the lentil and vegetable mixture and blend until smooth. Transfer the mixture to a large bowl.

Recipes

12. Slowly, with wet hands, stir in the bread crumbs, ¼ cup at a time, to the lentil mixture and mix with your hand until firm.
13. Place mixture in the refrigerator for about 30 minutes.
14. After 30 minutes, take the mixture and make small balls. Place each ball in a baking dish until you have used up all of the mixture.
15. Sprinkle with 1 tbs oil. Place in the oven for 20 minutes covered and then another 20 minutes uncovered.
16. Remove from oven
17. When they are browned, transfer the meatballs to the pan with marinara sauce and dip for a few minutes.
18. Serve on whole wheat spaghetti, garnish with chopped parsley.
19. Enjoy!

41. Millet Burger

Serves: 4
Preparation time: 10 minutes
Cooking time: 30 minutes

Ingredients

1 cup millet
4 cups water
2 tbs coconut oil
2 onions
1 clove garlic, peeled and minced
1 cup carrots
1 tsp Himalayan salt
1 tsp dill
1/4 cup parsley
1/4 cup sunflower seeds
1/2 cup rice, cooked (see recipe # 50)
1 tbs mustard

Recipes

Instructions:

1. Preheat oven to 350 degrees F (180 degree C)
2. On a pan, toast sunflower seeds
3. Rinse millet.
4. Place millet in a pot with 4 cups water. Bring to a boil for 1 minute. Reduce heat and simmer until all water is absorbed. Cover and set aside.
5. In a pan, sauté onions and garlic for 3 minutes.
6. Grate carrots and add to onions and garlic
7. In a separate bowl, mix salt, dill, parsley, toasted sunflower seeds, cooked rice.
8. Add vegetables and millet to bowl Continue mixing.
9. Make patties and place on baking paper in oven for 20-30 minutes.
10. Serve on whole wheat bun with mustard.
11. Enjoy!

42. Mediterranean Burger

Serves: 4
Preparation time: 24 hours
Cooking time: 20 minutes

Ingredients

1 cup sprouted green lentils
1 cup almonds
1 cup cashews
1/2 cup flax seeds
1/4 cups sesame seeds
1 cup parsley
1 tbs lemon juice
3 garlic cloves, minced
1 tsp cumin
1 tsp Himalayan salt
2 tbs coconut oil

Instructions:

1. Soak lentils in water for 8 hours. Wash and drain.
2. Wrap lentils in a damp paper towel, allow to sprout for 24 hours.
3. Soak almonds and cashews in water overnight.
4. Preheat oven to 350 degrees F (180 degree C)
5. Grind flax seeds
6. Place sprouted lentils, cashews, almonds, flax seeds, sesame seeds, parsley, lemon juice, garlic, cumin, salt and oil in the blender. Blend to smooth consistency.
7. Create patties with damp hands.
8. Place on baking paper on a baking sheet in oven for 20 minutes.
9. Serve on whole wheat bun with avocado or tahini (see recipe # 16).
10. Enjoy!

43. Lady Fingers and Tofu

Serves: 4
Preparation time: 5 minutes
Cooking time: 7 minutes

Ingredients

2 cups lady fingers
1 onion
1 cup firm tofu
6 garlic cloves
6 tomatoes
1 tsp black pepper
1 tbs cumin
1 tsp turmeric
1 tsp Himalayan salt
1 tbs coconut oil

Instructions:

1. Wash lady fingers and remove stems. Allow to dry in the sun.
2. Chop onion, mince garlic, dice tofu and chop tomatoes.
3. Heat oil in a wok or pan. Add onion, garlic tomatoes, spices and tofu.
4. Stir fry for 5 minutes.
5. Add lady fingers and bring to boil for 2 minutes. Lower heat and simmer partially covered for 1 hour.
6. Serve on brown rice (see recipe # 50).
7. Enjoy!

Breakfast

44. Healthy Pancakes

Serves: 4
Preparation time: 5 minutes
Cooking time: 5 minutes

Ingredients

1 cup spelt flour
1/2 cup bean flour
2 tbs wheat germ
2 tbs baking powder
1 pinch Himalayan salt
1/2 tsp cinnamon
1 - 1 1/2 cups almond milk
1 tbs coconut oil
1/4 cup raisins

Instructions:

1. Place flours, wheat germ, baking powder, salt and cinnamon in a bowl. Mix together.
2. In another bowl combine milk and oil together.
3. Gently poor the wet ingredients onto the dry ingredients. Add raisins.
4. Heat pan lightly brushed with coconut oil.
5. Pour batter onto pan. Spread batter with back of spoon to make pancake round and thin.
6. Cook until bubbling. Turn over. Remove when ready onto a paper towel and allow to cool.
7. Brush the pan with a little oil and go over the step above for each pancake.
8. Serve with sugar free organic jam of your choice.
9. Enjoy!

45. Tofu Shakshuka

Serves: 4
Preparation time: 5 minutes
Cooking time: 20 minutes

Ingredients

16 oz firm tofu
1 tbs coconut oil
1 clove garlic
1 onion
1 bell pepper
4 cups tomatoes, chopped
2 tbsp tomato paste
1 tsp chilli powder
1 tsp cumin
1 tsp paprika
1/2 tsp black pepper
1 pinch Himalayan salt

Instructions:

1. Chop onion, bell pepper, tomatoes, dice tofu and mince garlic. Heat oil in pan. Add chopped onion, sauté for a minute. Add garlic and continue to sauté for 1 minute.
2. Add the bell pepper, sauté for 5 minutes over medium heat.
3. Add tomatoes, tofu and tomato paste to mixture. Stir. Reduce heat to a simmer.
4. Add spices and stir for minutes.
5. Add salt and pepper and cayenne pepper if used (spicy).
6. Cover the pan. Allow mixture to simmer for 10-15 minutes.
7. Serve with toasted whole wheat pita bread.
8. Enjoy!

Recipes

46. Porridge

Serves: 4
Preparation time: 5 minutes
Cooking time: 5-7 minutes

Ingredients

1/2 cup oat groats
1/2 cup barley groats
2 cups almond milk

Instructions:

1. Place groats in a coffee bean blender.
2. Blend until semi smooth.
3. Add almond milk
4. Place in a pan and cook for 5 minutes.
5. Serve and enjoy!

Recipes

47. Oat and Seed Breakfast

Serves: 2
Preparation time: 5 minutes

Ingredients

1 cup oat meal
1 tbs chia seeds
1 tbs sunflower seeds
1 tbs pumpkin seeds
1 tbs flax seeds
2 cups almond milk

Instructions:

1. Add all ingredients into a bowl.
2. Serve and enjoy!

Recipes

48. Green Smoothie

Serves: 2
Preparation time: 5 minutes

Ingredients

1 pear
1 green apple
3 dates (seeded)
2 stalks celery
2 kale leaves
3 spinach leaves
4 twigs parsley
5 almonds
1 tbs clorella
1 tbs freshly squeezed lemon juice
2 tbs oat meal
1 cup ice cubes

Instructions:

1. Add all ingredients into a blender.
2. Blend until smooth. You may wish to add some water to make juice more fluid.
3. Serve and enjoy!

49. "Milk" Shake

Serves: 2
Preparation time: 5 minutes

Ingredients

1 red apple
1 banana
3 tbs oats
3 tbs sesame seed paste
1 cup almond milk
4 cubes ice

Instructions:

1. Place all ingredients in a blender.
2. Blend until smooth
3. Serve and enjoy!

Recipes

Basics

50. Brown Rice/Barley

Serves: 4
Preparation time: 2 hours
Cooking time: 45 minutes

Ingredients

1 cup brown Basmati rice or whole grain barley
1 pinch Himalayan salt (optional)

Instructions:

1. Take a cup of grains (barley or rice). Throughly rinse and cover with water to soak for 2 hours.
2. After soaking, drain the water.
3. Place rice in a pot and cover with three cups of water (for every one cup of rice) and salt.
4. Cover and bring to boil for 5 minutes. Reduce heat to a simmer until all the water is absorbed (approximately 40 minutes). Remove from heat,

still covered and allow to stand for 15 minutes. Enjoy!

51. Brown Rice with Black Lentils

Serves: 4
Preparation time: 2 hours
Cooking time: 45 minutes

Ingredients

1 cup brown Basmati rice
1 pinch Himalayan salt (optional)
1 cup Black lentils

Instructions:

1. Rinse lentils.
2. Take a cup of brown rice. Throughly rinse and cover with water to soak for 2 hours.
3. After soaking, drain the water.
4. Place rice and lentils in a pot and cover with four cups of water (for every one cup of rice and lentils) and salt.

5. Cover and bring to boil for 5 minutes. Reduce heat to a simmer until all the water is absorbed (approximately 40 minutes). Remove from heat, still covered and allow to stand for 15 minutes.
6. Enjoy!

Deserts

52. Healthy Vegan Winter Carrot Cake

Carrots are an exceptionally healthy vegetable. They have been proven to reduce cholesterol, and reduce the risk of a heart attack. Carrots are rich in potassium and thus reduce blood pressure, they are rich in antioxidants and support a healthy immune system - which is great for the winter. They are also great for weight loss due to their high fiber and low energy content and they reduce blood sugar levels as well. They are also super tasty and even improve eyesight! Carrots are truly a great vegetable!

Preparation time: 15 minutes
Cooking time: 50 minutes

Ingredients

3 1/2 cups grated carrots
1 1/2 cups whole wheat flour
1 1/2 tsp baking powder
1/2 tsp baking soda
1/2 tsp Himalayan salt
2 tsp cinnamon
1/2 tsp nutmeg
3 tbs freshly ground flax seeds mixed with 9 tbs water
1/2 cup coconut oil
1 1/2 tsp of liquid stevia extract
1 cup raisins
1/2 cup chopped walnuts

Instructions:

1. Preheat oven to 350 degree F (180 degree C)
2. Lightly spread some coconut oil on baking tray
3. In a small bowl, mix ground flaxseeds with 9 tbs water and allow to stand
4. In a large mixing bowl, mix flour, baking powder, baking soda, salt, cinnamon and nutmeg
5. Using an electric mixer, mix together flaxseed solution, coconut oil and stevia for 1 minute and then add flour mixture.
6. Mix together until smooth
7. Stir carrots, raisins, and walnuts into the mixture with a wooden spoon
8. Pour mixture into baking tray and bake for 50 minutes, or until a toothpick will come out clean if stayed in the cake centre.
9. Remove cake from oven and allow to cool for 1 hour
10. Serve and Enjoy!

Recipes

53. Raw Tasty Vegan Apple Pie

Apples are great for weight loss since they are rich in phytonutrients and in fiber that help regulate blood sugar levels and keep you feeling full for longer. This is a healthy apple pie. You can make it sugar free by exchanging the maple syrup with stevia.

Preparation time: 15 minutes

Ingredients - Base

1 tbs freshly ground flax seeds mixed with 3 tbs water
3 cups walnuts

2 tbs coconut oil
1 1/2 tsp baking powder
5 dates, seeded
1 cup natural sugar free jam of your choice

Ingredients - Filling

3 cups Granny Smith apples
3 tbs coconut butter
4 tbs maple syrup
1 tbs lemon juice
2 tsp cinnamon

Instructions:

1. Grind flaxseeds and place them in a small bowl, add 3 tbs water to the flaxseeds and allow to stand
2. Grind walnuts in a food processor, add the coconut oil and dates and grind again until smooth.
3. With a spoon, slowly mix in flaxseed solution
4. Press the nut, date and flaxseed mixture on the base of a round baking tray.

5. Smoothly top nut mixture with jam
6. Peel and thinly slice apples in a crescent shape. Place in a bowl.
7. Add maple syrup, lemon juice and cinnamon into bowl and gently stir together not breaking apples. Allow mixture to stand until apples become softer (about 5 minutes).
8. Neatly place apples on jam in the shape of a fan until whole cake is covered.
9. Place in refrigerator for 20 minutes before serving.
10. Serve and Enjoy!

Bread

54. Yeast Free Wholemeal Spelt & Walnut Bread

A healthy, yeast free wholemeal bread that's easy and simple to make. Spelt is one of the oldest cultivated crops in human history and is believed to have first been used 9,000 years ago. Spelt is closely related to wheat but is more nutritious than other forms of wheat don't have. Spelt is rich in B vitamins, zinc, magnesium, copper, phosphorous, selenium, copper as well as protein and fiber making it a great health promoting food.

Serves: 4
Preparation time: 10 minutes
Baking time: 50-60 minutes

Ingredients

1 cup walnuts
1tbs coconut oil to oil baking tray
4 cups whole grain spelt flour
1 1/2 tsp Himalayan salt
2 cups warm water or warmed almond milk
1 tsp baking powder
1 1/4 tsp baking soda
2 tbs molasses
1 tbs sunflower seeds
1 tbs pumpkin seeds
1 tsp black sesame seeds
1 tsp chia seeds

Instructions:

1. Preheat oven to 370 degrees F (190 degree C)
2. Spread walnuts on an English cake baking tray (preferably made from pyrex or stainless steel) and place in the oven to roast for 7-10 minutes.

Recipes

    Remove from oven and allow walnuts to cool. Chop into medium sized pieces.
3. Lightly spread coconut oil on baking tray
4. In a bowl, tip the flour, roasted chopped walnuts, salt, and baking soda. Mix
5. Slowly add the water and molasses to the dry mixture and mix together with your hands.
6. Place the mixture into oiled baking dish.
7. In a small bowl mix all seeds together and spread evenly on the bread dough mixture in baking dish
8. Place in oven and bake for 50-60 minutes
9. Remove bread from baking tray and allow to cool on a rack.
10. While cooling, brush bread with olive oil to make it softer.
11. Makes an excellent breakfast toped with almond seed paste.
12. Enjoy!

Bonus Recipes

55. Jerusalem Artichoke

A great tasting quick meal that supports a healthy gut bacteria allowing easier weight loss and optimal health.

Serves: 4
Preparation time: 15 minutes
Cooking time: 30 minutes

Ingredients

2 cups whole wheat pasta of your choice.
2 onions
3 garlic cloves, sliced
2 garlic cloves minced
2.2 pounds Jerusalem artichoke
1 tbs coconut oil
1 tbs turmeric

1 tsp ground rye
1 pinch Himalayan salt (optional)
1 pinch black pepper
3 tbs chopped parsley

Instructions:

1. Prepare pasta according to package instructions. Drain and rinse. Set aside.
2. Roast pine kernels for 2 minutes in a pan until lightly roasted. Set aside
3. Peel, wash and slice Jerusalem artichoke.
4. Place in a pot and cover with water. Add garlic to pot. Bring to boil for 1 minute.
5. Reduce heat and simmer for 20-30 minutes (until tender). Drain water. Remove from pot and set aside to cool.
6. Chop onions.
7. Heat oil in the pot. Add onions and minced garlic. Sauté for 2 minutes. Add artichokes and sauté for 1 minute. Add pasta, parsley, pine kernels and seasonings to mixture. Heat for 3 minutes.
8. Enjoy!

56. Miso Soup

Miso is a wonderful source of phytonutrient antioxidants and a very good source of manganese, copper, zinc and phosphorus as well as a good source of protein and dietary fiber. This makes miso have powerful anti cancer and heart protecting attributes. Miso also supports a healthy gut microbiota due to its fermentation process promoting optimal health and easier weight loss.

Serves: 4
Preparation time: 20 minutes
Cooking time: 60 minutes

Recipes

Ingredients

1 parsley root
1 celery root
1 stalk celery
3 carrots
1 onion
12 cups water
1/2 cup wakame seaweed
4 shiitake mushrooms
3 garlic cloves, sliced
1 handful bean sprouts
1/2 cup brown miso paste
1/2 cup cold water
1/2 pack firm tofu

Instructions:

1. Soak seaweed and mushrooms in water for 15 minutes. Wash, drain and set aside.
2. Wash and dice all vegetables.

Recipes

3. Place all vegetables in a pot and add the water. Bring to boil for one minute.
4. reduce heat and cook for 30 minutes on medium heat.
5. Add garlic, mushrooms and seaweed. Cook for 30 more minutes and remove from heat.
6. In a separate bowl blend the miso paste with the cold water. Add to the pot.
7. Place some bean sprouts and cubed tofu pieces in each serving bowl. Top with the soup.
8. Enjoy!

Recipes

57. Healthy Vegan Cholent Stew

A healthy, celebrational winter dish to serve when family and friends come together. This popular comfort dish was first mentioned in 1180 in Vienna, Austria. There are many recipes for cholent and ingredients vary according to the geographic regions.

Serves: 6
Preparation time: 12 hours
Cooking time: 8 hours

Ingredients

2 cups of white beans (with some red kidney beans if you like)
1 1/2 cups wholegrain barley (or wholegrain rice)
2 cups small black lentils
4 onions cut into 4
8 potatoes peeled and cut into chunks
Water or for more flavour use my vegan soup stock (see recipe #6)
1 tbs paprika
1 tbs turmeric
3 dates or 2 tbs of molasses
Pinch of Himalayan salt
Pinch of black pepper

Instructions:

1. Soak the white beans and barley seeds in water overnight. Wash beans and seeds and place them in an ovenproof pot.

2. Add to the pot the lentils, onions, potatoes, and spices.
3. Preheat oven to 200 degree F (100 degree C)
4. Cover the ingredients with water or vegan stock. Bring to boil and remove from heat. Stir.
5. Remove seeds from dates and add whole dates into the pot.
6. Cover pot and place in oven for 6-8 hours (the longer, the better), making sure there are enough liquids in the pot.
7. Serve and Enjoy!

Recipes

58. Mushrooms Stuffed With Macadamia Creme

Serves: 4
Preparation time: 15 minutes
Cooking time: 20 minutes

Ingredients

12 big forest mushrooms of any kind
3 cups macadamia nuts
6 dried tomatoes
1/2 cup spinach leaves, washed
4 garlic cloves
2 tbs olive oil
1 tsp Himalayan salt
1 pinch of black pepper

Recipes

Instructions:

1. Preheat oven to 350 degree F (180 degree C)
2. Gently wipe mushrooms clean with kitchen paper
3. Remove the mushroom leg from the base of the mushroom
4. Place macadamia nuts in food processor and grind. Add tomatoes, spinach leaves, garlic, olive oil, salt and pepper. Grind and mix until smooth.
5. Fill mushrooms with macadamia mixture.
6. Place mushrooms on a baking tray and bake for 20 minutes in oven.
7. Serve and Enjoy!

59. Quinoa Patties

Serves: 4
Preparation time: 10 minutes
Cooking time: 40 minutes

Ingredients

1/2 cup quinoa
1/2 cup yellow or green lentils
1 small pumpkin or squash
1 tbs coconut oil
1 tbs sesame seed paste
1 tsp cumin
1/2 tsp paprika
Pinch of Himalayan salt
Pinch of pepper

Instructions:

1. Preheat oven to 350 degree F (180 degree C)
2. Cube the pumpkin and place in then oven on a baking tray. Bake for 20 minutes.
3. Cook the lentils in 2 cups of boiling water for 10 minutes covered. After 10 minutes, add quinoa to the pot and cook the lentils and quinoa together for 10 minutes more. Remove from heat and leave to stand covered.
4. When the pumpkin is baked, remove from oven and mash with a fork.
5. Add the mashed pumpkin to the quinoa and lentil pot along with all of the other ingredients.
6. Allow mixture to cool enough to make patties.
7. Place patties on baking paper in the oven.
8. Bake for 10 minutes and turn over. Bake for another 10 minutes.
9. Serve and Enjoy!

Recipes

60. Vegan Banana Muffins

Serves: 4
Preparation time: 15 minutes
Cooking time: 20 minutes

Ingredients

3 bananas
1 1/2 cups whole wheat flour
1/2 cup oatmeal
1/2 cup raisins or any other dried fruit of your choice cut up the size of raisins
1 1/2 tsp baking powder
1/2 tsp baking soda
1/4 cup ground almonds
1 tsp ground cinnamon
1/4 teaspoon nutmeg
1/3 cup maple syrup/ agave or use 1/3 tsp stevia extract

1 tsp natural vanilla extract
1/2 cup coconut milk
4 tbs coconut oil

Instructions:

1. Preheat oven to 350 degree F (180 degree C)
2. Line 12 cup muffin pan with natural paper liners (If You Care Baking Cups)
3. Place the raisins in a cup and cover with hot water. Let to stand for a few minutes to plump and then drain excess water from raisins.
4. Chop bananas into small pieces.
5. In a bowl, stir together the whole wheat flour, oatmeal, baking powder, baking soda, cinnamon, nutmeg and ground almond flour.
6. Add oil, vanilla extract, coconut milk, maple syrup or stevia and raisins. Mix together using a wooden spoon.
7. Spoon mixture into muffin cups so they are about 2/3 full

Recipes

8. Place in oven and bake for 20-25 minutes until the muffins have browned and a toothpick comes out clean when inserted into the middle.
9. Remove from oven and allow to cool in the pan before removing from cups.
10. Serve and Enjoy!

Recipes

61. Tomato Soup

Tomatoes are a treasure box of antioxidant nutrients and have a unique phytonutrient composition. As a result, they provide critical protection against cancer and support a healthy cardiovascular system. The lycopene even protects our bones. Go for natural tomatoes rather than canned varieties.

Serves: 4
Preparation time: 10 minutes
Cooking time: 40 minutes

Ingredients

1 tbs coconut oil
1 onion
1 fennel

3 tbs uncooked brown rice
1 kg tomatoes
3 cups water
1 cup Shiitake mushrooms
3 tbs tomato paste
3 tbs tarragon
1 tsp fennel seeds
1/2 tsp stevia
Pinch of Himalayan salt
Pinch of pepper
1/4 cup red wine

Instructions:

1. Place the tomatoes in a pot and cover with water. Bring to boil and remove from heat. Peel tomatoes and cube them.
2. In the pot, heat coconut oil. Add onions and fennel. Stir fry for 5-8 minutes. Add the rice and continue to stir fry for 2 more minutes.
3. Mix in the chopped tomatoes to the pot.

4. Add the water with the whole Shiitake mushrooms to the pot. Add the tomato paste, tarragon, fennel seeds, stevia, Himalayan salt and pepper.
5. Bring to boil for 2 minutes. Lower the heat and cover. Cook for 25 minutes.
6. Remove mushrooms from pot. Add wine and cook for 5-8 minutes longer.
7. Serve and Enjoy!

Recipes

62. Healthy Vegan Birthday Chocolate Cake

Birthdays can be very exciting occasions especially for children. It provides them with pleasant memories and makes them the center of attention for the day highlighting the importance of self-love. Therefore, it is important to celebrate in a special way without compromising their health. This cake is one I have been using for years for each of my children (with slightly different toppings for each). Enjoy!

Serves: 15
Preparation time: 15 minutes
Cooking time: 40 minutes

Ingredients For The Cake

1/4 cup natural pecans
9 dried organic apricots
9 organic dates
3 cups whole meal rye flour
1/2 cup organic cocoa powder
1/2 cup coconut oil
1 tsp baking powder
1/2 tsp baking soda
2 cups water
1/2 cup maple syrup
2 tbs freshly squeezed lemon juice
pinch of salt
2 tsp natural vanilla extract
1/2 cup coconut milk
1/3 tsp stevia extract
100% chocolate bits

Ingredients For The Topping

3 cups whole cocoa powder
2 tbs coconut oil

Recipes

6 tbs maple syrup
6 tbs organic peanut butter
1 tsp vanilla extract
1/4 cup sugar free almond milk
1/3 tsp stevia extract
100% chocolate bits

Instructions:

1. Preheat oven to 350 degree F (180 degree C)
2. Place pecans in a blender and blend until they form a smooth consistency similar to flour. Place in a large mixing bowl.
3. Remove pits from dates. Chop apricots and dates into small pieces and place in a blender. Blend until the dried fruit are finely chopped. Add to the large mixing bowl.
4. Add the flour, cocoa, baking powder, baking soda and coconut oil to the mixing bowl and mix.
5. Add water, lemon juice, maple syrup, vanilla extract, chocolate chips and stevia. Mix until you have a smooth consistency. You may use a hand mixer for this.

Recipes

6. Lightly spread some coconut oil inside your desired cake pan.
7. Pour mixture into the baking pan and bake for 40 minutes, or until a toothpick will come out clean if stuck in the cake centre.
8. In the meantime prepare the cake topping: In the mixing bowl mix all topping ingredients except chocolate bits together using the hand mixer creating a smooth mixture. Add chocolate bits.
9. Remove cake from oven after 40 minutes and spread topping mixture on the cake.
10. To keep the cake healthy you may decorate it with strawberries, flowers and special candles. You can also add a printed edible photo to make your cake special and remove it before the cake is consumed.
11. Allow the cake to cool for at least one hour before serving, overnight is also fine.
12. Serve and Enjoy!

63. Healthy Wholegrain Vegan Pizza

A great way to transform an unhealthy food into a healthy alternative. Enjoy!

Serves: 4
Preparation time: 25 minutes
Backing time: 40 minutes

Ingredients For The Pizza

1 tbs dried yeast
1 1/2 cups whole grain flour of your choice
1/3 cup cornflour
1/2 cup hot water
Pinch of Himalayan salt
Dash of pepper

Recipes

Ingredients For The Cheese

1/4 cup natural raw cashews or macadamia nuts
1 cup hot water
3 tbs tapioca
1 tbs dry yeast
1 tsp freshly squeezed lemon juice
1/2 tsp garlic powder
Pinch of Himalayan salt
Dash of pepper

Ingredients For The Pizza Topping

3/4 cup organic tomato sauce
1 small red onion thinly sliced
5 button mushrooms thinly sliced
1/4 cup seeded olives
1 1/2 tsp dreid oregano
1/4 cup baby basil leaves

Instructions:

1. Soak cashews in water overnight. Drain. (you can also boil them until soft)
2. In a large mixing bowl, place the dried yeast, the whole grain flour, cornflour and mix together with a spoon. Add water and spices and mix together with your hands
3. Brush the dough with olive oil and leave in mixing bowl. Cover bowl with a towel and leave to rest for 20 minutes.
4. Preheat oven to 480 degree F (250 degree C)
5. In a blender, grind tapioca until it forms flour. Add cashews, hot water, yeast, lemon juice, garlic powder, salt and pepper and blend until smooth.
6. Pour into a sauce pan and cook for 10 minutes, while stirring make sure there are no nut pieces and the texture is smooth. You may need to use a hand blender to reach this consistency.
7. Slowly, while cooking, the mixture will become cheesy like. Stir for 2 more minutes until firm.
8. Place nut cheese in the refrigerator until pizza dough is ready.

9. Take dough and hit it so that all air from its centre is removed.
10. Spread the dough out to form a thin circular shape with rolled up borders. Brush borders with olive oil.
11. Spread tomato sauce on thin dough, cover with nut cheese, and spread thinly sliced vegetables over the pizza evenly.
12. Bake pizza n the lowest place in the oven for 15-20 minutes
13. Cover with spices and basil leaves
14. Serve and Enjoy!

64. Healthy Vegan Apple Crumble

Such a great, easy and healthy desert to make Enjoy!

Serves: 15
Preparation time: 15 minutes
Cooking time: 60 minutes

Ingredients For The Cake

5 Apples peeled and sliced into thin slices (I recommend using 3 McIntosh apples with 2 Granny Smith apples)
1 1/2 tsp cinnamon
2 tbs maple syrup
1/2 cup raisins
Juice from 1 freshly squeezed lemon

Recipes

Ingredients For The Crumble

1 cup wholegrain spelt flour
1/2 cup coconut butter
6 tbs maple syrup
1/3 tsp stevia extract

Instructions:

1. Preheat oven to 350 degree F (180 degree C)
2. In a mixing bowl mix together apples, cinnamon, raisins and lemon juice.
3. Transfer apple mixture into an oiled baking dish
4. Mix the crumble materials together with your hands until forms a crumble.
5. Spread the crumble on top of the apple mixture.
6. Place in oven for 1 hour.
7. Serve hot with scoop of vegan banana ice cream which can be made with just one ingredient - bananas, frozen and then blended to form a smooth texture!
8. Enjoy!

65. Healthy Vegan Energy Roll

When you need some energy during the day, here is a great nutritious snack to pick you up quickly. Great for adults and children alike! Enjoy!

Serves: 6
Preparation time: 15 minutes

Ingredients

3 tbs freshly ground flaxseeds
1 pack dates
1/2 cup coconut oil
1/4 cup maple syrup
1/4 cup pumpkin seeds
1/4 cup sunflower seeds
1/4 cup pistachios hulled and chopped

Recipes

1/4 cup chopped walnuts
1 tbs freshly squeezed lemon juice

Instructions:

1. In a small bowl, mix ground flaxseeds with 3 tbs water and allow to stand.
2. Deseed the dates and chop roughly. Place on the side.
3. In a pan, mix coconut oil with the maple syrup. Add the dates.
4. Cook until the mixture becomes mushy. Remove from heat.
5. Add flaxseed mixture to the pan and stir quickly.
6. Add the seeds and chopped walnuts, pistachios and lemon juice to the pan. Mix together.
7. Remove from pan to a sheet of baking paper. Create a roll the size of a sushi roll, you can use a sushi roller for this.
8. Once rolled, sprinkle some coconut flakes on top and place in the refrigerator for 10 minutes.

Recipes

9. When roll is hard, slice it into pieces.
10. Serve as an energy snack, great for kids and adults alike.
11. Enjoy!

Recipes

66. Lady Fingers and Chickpea Stew

Ladyfingers are the best solution for constipation. They are rich in fiber, make you feel full for longer and are packed with antioxidants, vitamins and minerals!

Serves: 6
Preparation time: 35 minutes
Cooking time: 50 minutes

Ingredients

1 cup chickpeas
3 cups water
1 tbs coconut oil
5 small onions
2 cloves garlic
4 medium tomatoes

Recipes

1 tbs freshly squeezed lemon juice
1 1/2 cups tomato juice
2 cups lady fingers (or zucchini)
1 tbs chopped oregano
Pinch of salt
pinch of black pepper

Instructions:

1. Soak chickpeas in water overnight, drain.
2. Toss ladyfingers in 1/2 cup vinegar and set aside for 30 minutes (to prevent it from becoming slimy)
3. Heat coconut oil in pan. Add onions (whole if they are small enough), and garlic. Fry for 5 minutes.
4. Peel and chop tomatoes.
5. Add tomatoes, chickpeas, lemon juice and tomato juice to pan. Cover and simmer for 30 minutes.
6. Rinse ladyfingers thoroughly from vinegar.
7. Add lady fingers to pan and cook for 20 more minutes (if using zucchini, cook for 10 minutes)
8. Add oregano, salt and pepper.
9. Serve with wholegrain brown Basmati rice.
10. Serve and Enjoy!

Recipes

Notes

Recipes

Notes

Recipes

Notes

Recipes

Notes

Recipes

Notes

Recipes

Notes

Recipes

Notes

Recipes

Notes

Recipes

Notes

Recipes

Notes

All Books By Galit Goldfarb

1. The Guerrilla Diet & Lifestyle Program - Wage War On Weight and Poor Health and Learn To Thrive In The Modern Jungle.
2. How to Achieve Success and Happiness series:
   1. The 6 Principle Strategy for Creating a Successful & Happy Life: Book # 1: The Basics Everyone Needs to Know
   2. The 6 Principle Strategy for Creating a Successful & Happy Life: Book # 2: How to Create Peace of Mind
   3. The 6 Principle Strategy for Creating a Successful & Happy Life: Book # 3: How to Create Optimum Health
   4. The 6 Principle Strategy for Creating a Successful & Happy Life: Book # 4: How to Create Great Relationships
   5. The 6 Principle Strategy for Creating a Successful & Happy Life: Book # 5: How to Create Wealth
3. Best Way To Lose Weight - A Step-By-Step Guide to Lose Weight In A Month The Guerrilla Diet Way
4. 50 Best Recipes For Health and Weight Loss - The Guerrilla Diet Way

Made in the USA
Columbia, SC
27 June 2019